HK SPORT SCIENCE MONOGRAPH SERIES

Volume 8

Catastrophic Injuries in High School and College Sports

Frederick O. Mueller, PhD
National Center for Catastrophic Sports Injury Research

Robert C. Cantu, MD
Emerson Hospital, Concord, MA

Steven P. Van Camp, MD
President, American College of Sports Medicine, 1995-96

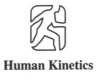

Human Kinetics

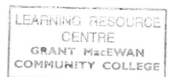

Library of Congress Cataloging-in-Publication Data

Mueller, Frederick O.
  Catastrophic injuries in high school and college sports /
  Frederick O. Mueller, Robert C. Cantu, Steven P. Van Camp.
    p. cm.
  Includes bibliographical references.
  ISBN 0-87322-674-7 (pbk.)
  1. Sports injuries.   2. College athletes--Wounds and injuries.
  3. High school athletes--Wounds and injuries.   4. Spinal cord-
  -Wounds and injuries.   5. Brain--Wounds and injuries.   I. Cantu,
  Robert C.   II. Van Camp, Steven P.   III. Title.
    [DNLM: 1. Athletic Injuries--in adolescence.   2. Athletic
  Injuries--in adulthood.   QT   261   M946c   1996]
  RD97.M84   1996
  617.1'027--dc20
  DNLM/DLC
  for Library of Congress   95-31210
                                                                  CIP

ISBN: 0-87322-674-7
ISSN: 0894-4229

Copyright © 1996 by Frederick O. Mueller, Robert C. Cantu, and Steven P. Van Camp

Tables 2.1, 2.2, 2.4, and 2.5 are from "Nontraumatic Sports Death in High School and College Athletes," by S. Van Camp et al., May 1995, *Medicine and Science in Sports and Exercise*, **27**(5), pp. 641-647. Copyright 1995. Reprinted with permission.

Acquisitions Editor: Richard A. Washburn; **Developmental Editor**: Elaine Mustain; **Assistant Editors**: Erin Cler, Chad Johnson; **Editorial Assistant**: Andrew Starr; **Copyeditor**: Sue Tyson; **Proofreader**: Kathy Bennett; **Production Manager**: Ernie Noa; **Typesetting and Text Layout**: Sandra Meier; **Layout Artist**: Denise Lowry; **Text Designer**: Judy Henderson; **Cover Designer**: Jody Boles; **Illustrator**: Nichole Barbuto; **Printer**: Versa Press

Printed in the United States of America

10   9   8   7   6   5   4   3   2   1

Human Kinetics
P.O. Box 5076, Champaign, IL 61825-5076
1-800-747-4457

Canada: Human Kinetics, Box 24040, Windsor, ON N8Y 4Y9
1-800-465-7301 (in Canada only)

Europe: Human Kinetics, P.O. Box IW14, Leeds LS16 6TR, United Kingdom
(44) 1132 781708

Australia: Human Kinetics, 2 Ingrid Street, Clapham 5062, South Australia
(08) 371 3755

New Zealand: Human Kinetics, P.O. Box 105-231, Auckland 1
(09) 523 3462

This book is dedicated
to all high school and college athletes
who suffered a catastrophic injury
during their participation in athletics,
and to the many sports medicine researchers
who are working to help reduce these injuries.
Hopefully this book will play a significant role
in reducing catastrophic injuries in sports.

Contents

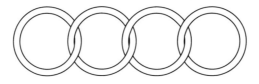

Introduction

Catastrophic sports injury research in high school and college sports in the United States, with the exception of football, is a recent phenomenon. Only within the past 10 to 15 years has any organized research been carried out in sports other than football, and the literature in female catastrophic athletic injuries is nonexistent.

Catastrophe, as defined by *Webster's Ninth New Collegiate Dictionary*, is the final event of the dramatic action of a tragedy—a momentous tragic event. Catastrophic athletic injuries, although comprising a small percentage of all catastrophic injuries, are tragic events affecting the lives of mostly young healthy individuals. For example, of the 2,500 new cases of paraplegia and the 1,050 new cases of quadriplegia in the United States each year, about 7% (175 paraplegia and 74 quadriplegia) are related to sports injury.

Of the 410,000 people who sustain brain injury each year, 17,600 are left with some type of permanent disability. About 10% of brain injuries are the result of sport or recreational activity. Approximately 142,568 people die as a result of injury each year. Injuries are the leading cause of death for children and young adults (under age 45) and are the fourth overall cause of death in the US.

Although the percentage of total deaths related to sport participation is low, these deaths are tragic events for which every possible step toward prevention should be taken. Before preventive measures can be effectively implemented, it is important to determine what types of injuries are most prevalent, who sustains the injuries, and why and where they occur.

An effort to answer these questions began in 1965 at the University of North Carolina-Chapel Hill (UNC-CH) with a research project to study catastrophic injuries in football. The success of this project in identifying factors related to catastrophic injuries led to rule changes in 1976 that eliminated initial contact with the head and face during blocking and tackling, developed standards for football helmet construction, and improved medical care and coaching methods.

In 1982, the National Center for Catastrophic Sports Injury Research (NCCSIR) was established at UNC-CH to expand the data collection to include women's sports and to expand the sports covered. These expansions were made because research based on reliable data is essential if progress is to be made in sport safety, because of the paucity of injury data in sports other than football, and because of the rapid expansion and total lack of injury data in women's sports. We based this book on data collected as a result of that decision.

Definition of Terms

For the purpose of this book, catastrophic injuries will generally be limited to high school and college sports for both female and male athletes although the chapter on football includes junior and senior high school athletes. Catastrophic is defined as any severe spine, spinal cord, or cerebral injury incurred in a school- or college-sponsored sport. It includes the following three divisions:

1. Fatal
2. Nonfatal—permanent functional disability
3. Serious—no permanent functional disability but severe injury. An example is a fractured cervical vertebra with complete recovery.

Catastrophic injuries will also be divided into direct and indirect as follows:

- *Direct*—injuries that result directly from participation in the sport. Examples are tackling in football or making a save in field hockey.
- *Indirect*—injuries caused by systemic failure as a result of exertion while participating in a sport activity or by a complication that is secondary to a nonfatal injury. Sudden cardiac death is an example of an indirect catastrophic injury.

Other terms used in the book are:

Incidence—the total number of injuries.

Prevalence—the percentage of the study population with a particular type of injury.

Injury rate—dividing the number of injured players by the total number of players will give an injury rate per 100,000 participants (or for whatever number selected). By dividing the number of players into the total number of injuries and multiplying by 100,000, an injury rate per 100,000 participants is established.

Athlete exposure—one athlete participating in one practice or game in which he or she is exposed to possible injury.

Data Collection

Data collection for the research presented in this book would not have been possible without a grant from the National Collegiate Athletic Association (NCAA), support from the American Football Coaches Association (AFCA), and the efforts of the National Federation of State High School Associations

(NFSHSA) and their 50 state associations. At the beginning of the study, and each subsequent year, coaches, athletic directors, executive officers of state and national athletic organizations, athletic trainers, a national newspaper clipping service, and professional associates of the authors were contacted to inform them that the research was in progress. Thus, the NCCSIR was informed annually of the occurrence of catastrophic injuries.

Upon receiving information concerning a possible catastrophic sports injury, contact was made by telephone, personal letter, and questionnaire with the injured player's coach, athletic director, or athletic trainer. Data collected included demographic information on the athlete (age, sex, playing experience, grade, height, weight), accident information (sport, game or practice, date, how accident happened, etc.), medical information (medical history, immediate and postaccident medical care, body part injured and type of injury, disability, autopsy report if available), and equipment involved in the accident (type of equipment, make and model, condition).

In addition to the information collected concerning the accident, medical information from the case physician was collected by the medical director of the NCCSIR. Accurate medical data are important when classifying injuries and making recommendations for prevention.

It should be noted that a limitation of the research is that there is no guarantee that the NCCSIR has 100% case ascertainment. No validity checks were made. Fatality data is easier to collect on a national level because fatalities receive so much attention. There is usually less attention paid to a disability injury, and always less attention paid to a serious injury.

All participation numbers were obtained from the NFSHSA in Kansas City, MO, and the NCAA in Overland Park, KS.

Book Organization

The remainder of the book will be organized in the following manner:

- Chapter 1 provides medical information about catastrophic head and neck injuries in sports. This chapter was written by Robert C. Cantu, M.D., medical director of the NCCSIR, a neurosurgeon, and the head of surgery and chief of sports medicine at Emerson Hospital in Concord, MA. Dr. Cantu is also the past president of the American College of Sports Medicine.
- Chapter 2 provides medical information and terms associated with sudden death in athletics and includes 10 years' worth of in-depth data (covering the period July 1983-June 1993) on sudden death in high school and college sports. This chapter was written by Steven P. Van Camp, M.D., an experienced cardiologist from San Diego, CA, who has also been involved in data collection with the NCCSIR. He is the current president of the American College of Sports Medicine.
- Chapter 3 examines the catastrophic injury experience of football players due to the sport's long history of injury data collection. Football fatality

data have been collected since 1931 and disability data from 1977. Data here include information collected prior to 1982.

- Chapter 4 treats the catastrophic injury experience in team sports other than football, including soccer, basketball, ice hockey, baseball, and lacrosse. This chapter will include 10 years' worth of data from the fall of 1982 to the spring of 1992, cause of injury, and case studies.
- Chapter 5 treats the catastrophic injury experience in sports involving individual competition, including gymnastics, swimming, wrestling, track and field, and cheerleading. This chapter will include 10 years' worth of data from the fall of 1982 to the spring of 1992, cause of injury, and case studies.
- Chapter 6 provides recommendations for the prevention of catastrophic injuries in high school and college athletics. Recommendations will be given for preparticipation exams, proper conditioning, medical care, prevention of heat stress, proper training of coaches, and supporting the decisions of referees. The final section of this chapter will include specific recommendations for each sport.

Chapter 1

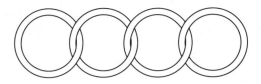

Catastrophic Head and Spine Injuries

The head and spine are unique in that their contents are incapable of regeneration. The brain and spinal cord cannot regrow lost cells, as can other organs of the body; thus injury to these structures takes on a singular importance. Whereas today virtually every major joint (ankle, knee, hip, elbow, shoulder) and most major organs can be replaced, either by artificial hardware or transplanted parts, the head and spine cannot be replaced: Their contents cannot be transplanted. The most complex and vital area of the body, the central nervous system (CNS), housed in the skull and spine, can recover from injury to cells, but once a cell or cells have died, no replacement is possible. With these sobering facts in mind, let us look at the etiology of catastrophic head and spine injury in general and as it specifically applies to different sports.

Etiology of Brain Injury

An understanding of the forces that produce skull and brain injuries requires an understanding of the following principles:

1. A forceful blow to the resting movable head usually produces maximum brain injury beneath the point of cranial impact (*coup* injury).
2. A moving head impacting against an unyielding object usually produces maximum brain injury opposite the site of cranial impact (*contrecoup* injury). Such lesions are most common at the tips and the undersurfaces of the frontal and temporal lobes.
3. If a skull fracture is present, the first two dictums do not pertain because the bone itself, displaced either transiently (linear skull fracture) or permanently (depressed skull fracture) at the moment of impact, may directly injure brain tissue.

With brain and spinal cord injuries, it is also essential to recognize that three types of stresses can be generated by an applied force: *compressive*, *tensile* (the opposite of compressive, sometimes called negative pressure), and *shearing* (a force applied parallel to a surface). Neural tissue can tolerate uniform tensile and compressive stresses fairly well but it tolerates shearing stresses very poorly.

The cerebrospinal fluid (CSF) acts as a shock absorber, cushioning and protecting the brain by converting focally applied external stresses to a more uniform compressive stress. Despite the presence of CSF, however, shearing stresses may still be imparted to the brain. If rotational forces are applied to the head, shearing forces will occur at those sites where rotational gliding is hindered. These areas are characterized by

- rough irregular surface contacts between the brain and skull, hindering smooth movement;
- dissipation of the cerebrospinal fluid between the brain and skull; and
- dura mater brain attachments impeding brain motion.

The first condition is most prominent in the frontal and temporal regions and explains why major brain contusions occur at these sites. The second condition explains the coup and contrecoup injuries. When the head is accelerated prior to impact, the brain lags toward the trailing surface, thus squeezing away protective CSF and allowing for the shearing forces to be maximal at this site. This brain lag actually thickens the layer of CSF under the point of impact, which explains the lack of coup injury in moving head injury. On the other hand, when the head is stationary prior to impact, there is neither brain lag nor disproportionate distribution of CSF, accounting for the absence of contrecoup injury and the presence of coup injury.

The scalp also has energy-absorbing properties. It requires 10 times more force to produce a skull fracture in a cadaveric head with the scalp in place than in one with the scalp removed. In addition, Newton's law that "force equals mass times acceleration" pertains in this situation. An athlete's head can sustain far greater forces without brain injury if the neck muscles are tensed at the moment of impact. In the relaxed state, the mass of the head is essentially its own weight. However, with the neck rigidly tensed, the mass of the head approximates the mass of the body.

Etiology of Cervical Spine Injury

The cervical spine is composed of seven vertebrae joined by multiple ligaments, intervening cartilages, and muscles. In the lateral view, it is curved, convex forward (*lordosis*). The ligaments, consisting of elastin and collagen, provide the primary stabilizing component of the cervical spine. Elastin fibers arranged in a parallel manner longitudinally allow the ligaments to stretch up to twice their length and yet return to their original length. The main ligaments are the anterior and posterior longitudinal, intertransverse and capsular, interspinal and supraspinal, and ligamentum flavum.

The muscle groups posterior to the spinal column are significantly greater than those anterior to it. Coupled with the fact that neck movement in flexion is limited by chin contact with the sternum (whereas extension is possible until the head strikes the posterior chest wall), this muscle disparity makes extension injuries potentially more serious than flexion injuries, given an equivalent amount of force. Thus, the spine is more resistant to flexion injury than extension injury.

External forces can flex, extend, rotate, or compress the spine. In flexion injury (see Figure 1.1), the anterior elements are compressed, causing anterior-wedging, vertebral body fracture, chip fracture, and occasionally anterior dislocations. The posterior elements are injured, which results in rupture of the posterior longitudinal, interspinal, and supraspinal ligaments and the ligamentum flavum. Occasionally, rupture of the posterior half of the disc is seen.

With an extension spine injury (whiplash) (see Figure 1.2, page 8), the anterior elements are disrupted and the posterior elements are compressed. This leads to rupture of the anterior longitudinal ligament and anterior disc, with posterior bony injury to the spinous processes, facets, and the neural arch.

A compression, or burst injury (see Figure 1.3, page 9), occurs with vertical loading of the spine, such as from a blow to the vertex with the neck flexed.

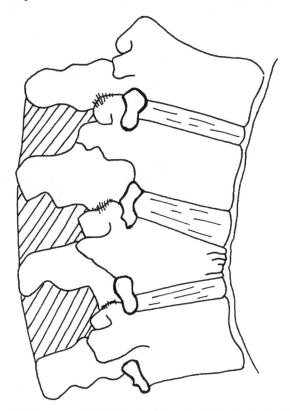

Figure 1.1 Flexion injury to the spine.

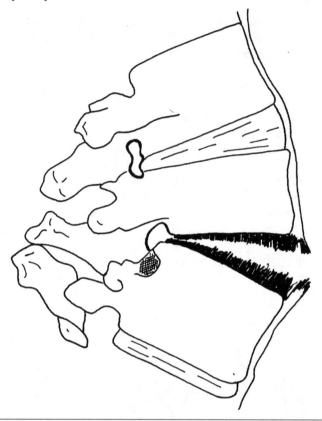

Figure 1.2 Extension injury to the spine.

This leads to vertebral end-plate fractures before the disc injury. At higher forces, the entire vertebra and disc may explode into the spinal canal. Analysis has shown this to be the major mechanism of cervical fracture or dislocation and quadriplegia, not only in football (e.g., spearing, butt blocking) but also in diving injuries and, increasingly, in (Canadian) ice hockey neck injuries (1, 2).

With the normal head-up posture, the cervical spine has a gentle lordotic curve, and forces transmitted to the head are largely dissipated in the cervical muscles. When the neck is flexed, however, the cervical spine becomes straight, with the vertebral bodies lined up under one another. The forces of impact to the vertex of the head are directly transmitted from one vertebra to the next. This allows for minimal dissipation of the impact forces in the neck muscles. If the impact force exceeds the strength of the bone, it compacts it at one or more levels. This results in a compression fracture. If the fractured vertebra malaligns and is driven back into the spinal cord, quadriplegia may result.

A combined flexion-rotation injury (see Figure 1.4, page 10) is most likely to result not only in a flexion injury, but also in anterior subluxation. Subluxation is usually found only in the presence of rotation and is more easily produced in flexion than in extension.

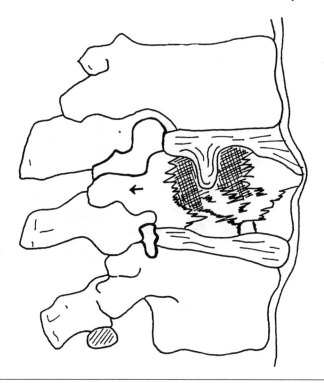

Figure 1.3   Compression (burst) injury to the spine. The arrow indicates direction of force.

Most cervical spine flexion, extension, and rotation injuries occur with head trauma, but it is important to realize that such injuries can result from other causes as well. Extension injury can occur with sudden acceleration forward, that is, a block or tackle from the rear. Flexion injury can occur with sudden deceleration, that is, when the force is delivered from the front. Neck fractures also may occur with sudden cranial acceleration of the lower torso or buttocks (as with a fall broken by landing on one's buttocks or by direct impact to the posterior cervical region by blunt trauma).

Types of Brain Injury

The types of brain injury seen in sports are concussion, postconcussion syndrome, intracranial hemorrhage, and second impact syndrome.

Concussion

What are the definitions and grades of severity of concussion? Consensus on the definition of concussion does not exist, making evaluation of the epidemiologic data extremely difficult. The Committee on Head Injury Nomenclature of the Congress of Neurological Surgeons has put forth a working definition of concussion that has gained general acceptance: "a clinical syndrome characterized by

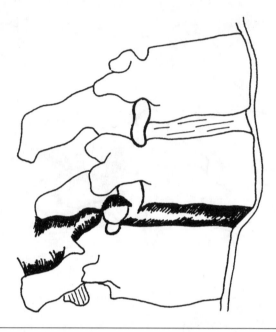

Figure 1.4   Flexion-rotation injury to the spine.

immediate and transient posttraumatic impairment of neural function, such as alteration of consciousness, disturbance of vision, equilibrium, etc. due to brain-stem involvement'' (3).

Maroon (1980), in attempting to simplify the clinical problem, divided concussion into three grades based on duration of unconsciousness: mild (no loss of consciousness), moderate (loss of consciousness under 5 min with retrograde amnesia), and severe (unconsciousness longer than 5 min) (4). Others have classified concussion according to duration of posttraumatic amnesia (5). As a team physician, I have seen many concussions. Most were mild, and posttraumatic amnesia, which helped me make the diagnosis, was usually present. Combining elements of the various definitions of concussion has afforded me an easy, practical, on-the-field grading scheme (see Table 1.1) (6).

Grade 1 (Mild) Concussion

The mild concussion is the most difficult to recognize and judge. The patient does not lose consciousness but suffers from impaired intellectual function, especially in remembering recent events and in assimilating and interpreting new information. Grade 1 concussion occurs most frequently (more than 90% of concussions) and often escapes medical attention (7). Players commonly are ''dinged'' or have their ''bell rung'' and continue playing. Dave Meggyesy, a professional football player-turned-author, described this condition: ''Your memory's affected, although you can still walk around and sometimes continue

Table 1.1   Severity of Concussion

Grade 1 (mild)	No *LOC; †PTA 30 min
Grade 2 (moderate)	LOC < 5 min or PTA > 30 min
Grade 3 (severe)	LOC ≥ 5 min or PTA ≥ 24 hr

*Loss of consciousness.

†Posttraumatic amnesia.

From Cantu RC: Guidelines to return to contact sports after cerebral concussion. PhysSportsmed 14:76, 1986 with permission.

playing. If you don't feel pain, the only way others know that you have been 'dinged' is when they realize you can't remember the plays'' (8).

Initial treatment of a mild concussion requires the player to be removed from the game and observed on the bench. After a sufficient period of time (which may be as short as 15 to 30 min), if the athlete has no headache, dizziness, or impaired concentration (including orientation to person, place, and time, as well as full recall of events that occurred just before the injury), return to the game may be considered (4, 7). Before such players are allowed to return, however, they should be asymptomatic not only at rest but also after demonstrating that they can move with their usual dexterity and speed during exertion. If an athlete has any symptoms during either rest or exertion, continued neurologic observation is essential.

Grade 2 (Moderate) Concussion

With moderate concussion (unconsciousness lasting less than 5 min), initial management should be the same as for Grade 3. The athlete should be removed from the game and evaluated by a neurologist at a medical facility. Here, though, clinical judgment may dictate that if the period of unconsciousness is brief and the athlete has no neck problems after regaining consciousness, removal on a fracture board may not be necessary.

Grade 3 (Severe) Concussion

It is not difficult to recognize a severe concussion (unconsciousness lasting 5 min or more). Initial treatment should be the same as the treatment for a suspected cervical spine fracture. The athlete should be transported on a fracture board, with head and neck immobilized, to a hospital with neurosurgical treatment facilities. All severe concussions should be admitted to check for possible intracranial bleeding (9, 10).

Postconcussion Syndrome

This syndrome consists of headache (especially with exertion), labyrinthine disturbance, fatigue, irritability, and impaired memory and concentration (11). Its true incidence is not known; however, it has been uncommon in my experience to last longer than a week or two. Persistence of symptoms reflects altered neurotransmitter function (11), usually correlates well with the duration of post-traumatic amnesia (12), and suggests that the athlete should be evaluated with a computerized tomography (CT) scan and neuropsychiatric testing. The athlete's return to competition should be deferred until all symptoms have abated and diagnostic studies are normal.

Intracranial Hemorrhage

The leading cause of death from athletic head injury is intracranial hemorrhage. There are four types of hemorrhage to which the examining trainer or physician must be alert in every instance of head injury: epidural hematoma, subdural hematoma, intracerebral hematoma, and subarachnoid hemorrhage. Because all four types of intracranial hemorrhage may be fatal, rapid, accurate initial assessment as well as appropriate follow-up is mandatory after an athletic head injury.

Epidural Hematoma

An epidural (or extradural) hematoma is usually the most rapidly progressing intracranial hemorrhage: It may reach a fatal size in 30 to 60 min. It is frequently associated with a fracture of the temporal bone and results from a tear of the artery supplying the covering (dura) of the brain. This hematoma accumulates inside the skull but outside the covering of the brain. The athlete may have a lucid interval, initially remaining conscious or regaining consciousness after the head trauma, before starting to experience increasing headache and progressive deterioration in the level of consciousness as the clot accumulates and the intracranial pressure increases.

This lesion will almost always declare itself within 1 to 2 hr from the time of injury. Usually the brain substance is free from direct injury; thus, if the clot is promptly removed surgically, full recovery is to be expected. Because this lesion is rapidly and universally fatal if missed, however, all athletes receiving a major head injury must be observed very closely during the ensuing several hours, and preferably the next 24 hr. This observation should be done at a facility where full neurosurgical services are immediately available.

Subdural Hematoma

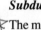

The most common fatal athletic head injury, a subdural hematoma occurs between the brain surface and the dura, and is thus located under the dura and directly on the brain. It often results from a torn vein running from the surface of the brain to the dura, but may also result from a torn venous sinus or even a small artery on the surface of the brain. With this injury, there is often associated injury to the brain tissue. If a subdural hematoma necessitates surgery in the first 24 hr, the mortality is high, due not to the clot itself but to the associated brain damage. With a subdural hematoma that progresses rapidly, the athlete usually does not regain consciousness, and the need for immediate neurosurgical evaluation is obvious.

Occasionally, the brain itself will not be injured, and a subdural hematoma may develop slowly over a perod of days to weeks. This chronic subdural hematoma, although often associated with headache, may initially cause a variety of very mild, almost imperceptible mental, motor, or sensory symptoms. Because its recognition and removal will lead to full recovery, it must always be suspected in an athlete who has previously sustained a head injury and who, days or weeks later, is "not quite right." A computerized axial tomography (CAT) scan of the head will definitely show such a lesion.

Intracerebral Hematoma

Intracerebral hematomas are not usually associated with an interval of lucidity and may be rapidly progressive. Here, the bleeding is into the brain substance itself, usually from a torn artery. An intracerebral hematoma may be caused by head trauma, but it may also result from the rupture of a congenital vascular lesion such as an aneurysm or arteriovenous malformation.

Death occasionally occurs before the injured athlete can be moved to a hospital. Because of the intense reaction such a tragic event precipitates among fellow athletes, family, students, and even the community at large, and because of the inevitable rumors that follow, it is imperative to obtain a complete autopsy in such an event to fully clarify the causative factors. Often the autopsy will reveal a congenital lesion that may indicate that the cause of death was other than presumed—and ultimately unavoidable. Only by such full, factual elucidation will inappropriate feelings of guilt in fellow athletes, friends, and family be assuaged.

Subarachnoid Hemorrhage

Subarachnoid hemorrhages are confined to the surface of the brain. Following head trauma, such bleeding is the result of disruption of the tiny surface brain vessels and is analogous to a bruise. As with the intracerebral hematoma, there is often brain swelling, and such a hemorrhage can also result from a ruptured cerebral aneurysm or arteriovenous malformation. Because bleeding is superficial, surgery is not usually required unless a congenital vascular anomaly is present.

Such a contusion of the brain usually causes headache and, not infrequently, an associated neurologic deficit, depending on the area of the brain involved. The irritative properties of the blood may also precipitate a seizure. If a seizure occurs in a head-injured athlete, it is important to roll the patient onto his or her side so that any blood or saliva will roll out of the mouth or nose and the tongue cannot fall back, obstructing the airway. If one has a padded tongue depressor or oral airway, it can be inserted between the teeth. (Under no circumstances should one insert one's fingers into the mouth of an athlete who is having a seizure, as the athlete could easily bite them off under the force of convulsions.) Usually such a traumatic seizure will last only for a minute or two. The athlete will then relax, and can be transported to the nearest medical facility.

Following any of the four types of intracranial hemorrhage, prophylactic anticonvulsant therapy with dilantin is usually given for 1 year. Because the chance of posttraumatic epilepsy is under 10% with a concussion or contusion, anticonvulsant therapy is given in these conditions only if late epilepsy actually occurs (13).

Second Impact Syndrome

Second impact syndrome (SIS), or the rapid brain swelling and herniation following a second head injury, is more common than previous reports in the medical literature have suggested (14-16). Between 1980 and 1993, the National Center for Catastrophic Sports Injury Research (NCCSIR) in Chapel Hill, North Carolina, identified 35 probable cases among football players alone. Autopsy or surgery and magnetic resonance imaging (MRI) findings confirmed 17 of these cases. An additional 18 cases probably are SIS, though they have not been conclusively documented with autopsy findings. Careful scrutiny excluded this diagnosis in 22 of 57 cases originally suspected.

SIS is not confined to football players, however. Reports of head injury among athletes in other sports almost certainly represent the syndrome but do not label it as such. Fekete (17), for example, described a 16-year-old high school hockey player who fell during a game, striking the back of his head on the ice. The boy lost consciousness and afterward complained of unsteadiness and headaches. While playing in the next game 4 days later, he was checked forcibly and again fell, striking his left temple on the ice. His pupils rapidly became fixed and dilated, and he died within 2 hr while in transit to a neurosurgical facility.

The autopsy report revealed occipital contusions of several days' duration, an edematous brain with a thin layer of subdural and subarachnoid hemorrhage, and bilateral herniation of the cerebellar tonsils into the foramen magnum. Though Fekete did not use the label SIS, the clinical course and autopsy findings in this case are consistent with the syndrome.

Such cases indicate that the brain is vulnerable to accelerative forces in a variety of contact and collision sports. Therefore, physicians who cover athletic events, especially those in which head trauma is likely, must understand SIS and be prepared to initiate emergency treatment.

Recognizing the Syndrome

What Saunders and Harbaugh (18) called the second impact syndrome of catastrophic head injury in 1984 was first described by Schneider (19) in 1973. The syndrome occurs when an athlete who sustains a head injury—often a concussion or worse injury, such as cerebral contusion—sustains a second head injury before symptoms associated with the first have cleared.

Typically, the athlete suffers postconcussional symptoms after the first head injury. These may include visual, motor, or sensory changes and difficulty with thought and memory processes. Before these symptoms resolve—which may take days or weeks—the athlete returns to competition and receives a second blow to the head.

The second blow may be remarkably minor, perhaps involving a blow to the chest, side, or back that merely snaps the athlete's head and indirectly imparts accelerative forces to the brain. The athlete usually remains standing for 15 seconds to a minute or so, and indeed often completes the play or walks off the field. But the athlete seems dazed, similar to someone suffering from a Grade 1 concussion (that is, without loss of consciousness) (6).

What happens in the next 15 seconds to several minutes sets this syndrome apart from a concussion or even a subdural hematoma: The athlete, conscious though stunned, quite precipitously collapses to the ground semicomatose with rapidly dilating pupils, loss of eye movement, and evidence of respiratory failure.

The pathophysiology of SIS is thought (18-20) to involve loss of autoregulation of the brain's blood supply. This loss of autoregulation leads to vascular engorgement within the cranium (6, 20), which in turn markedly increases the intracranial pressure and leads to herniation either of the medial surface (uncus) of the temporal lobe or lobes below the tentorium or herniation of the cerebellar tonsils through the foramen magnum. The usual time from second impact to brainstem failure is rapid, taking 2 to 5 min. Once brain herniation and brainstem compromise occur, coma, ocular involvement, and respiratory failure ensue precipitously. This demise occurs far more rapidly than that usually seen with an epidural hematoma.

Prevention Is Primary

For a catastrophic condition that has a mortality rate approaching 50% and a morbidity rate nearing 100%, prevention takes on the utmost importance. An athlete who is symptomatic from a head injury *must not* participate in contact or collision sport until all cerebral symptoms have subsided, and preferably not for at least 1 week thereafter. Whether it takes days, weeks, or months to reach the asymptomatic state, the athlete must *never* be allowed to practice or compete while exhibiting postconcussion symptoms.

Players and parents as well as the physician and medical team must understand this. Files of the NCCSIR include cases of young athletes who did not report their cerebral symptoms. Fearing they would not be allowed to compete and not knowing they were jeopardizing their lives, they played with postconcussional symptoms and tragically developed SIS.

Types of Spine Injuries

The same traumatic lesions that affect the brain—concussion, contusion, and the various types of hemorrhage—may also occur to the cervical spinal cord.

Fracture, Concussion, Contusion, Hemorrhage

Unlike with the head, where the subdural hematoma is the most common and lethal type of hemorrhage, the subdural hematoma is uncommon in the spine. Since I have been associated with the NCCSIR, there have been no spinal subdural hematomas. Instead, the intraspinal (within the cord) is the most common and epidural next most common type of hemorrhage. In addition, all spinal hemorrhages have been in the cervical region, and none have been seen in the thoracic or lumbar region.

The major concern with a cervical spinal injury is the possibility of an unstable fracture that may produce quadriplegia. In the NCCSIR registry, all cases of quadriplegia in the absence of spinal stenosis resulted from fracture dislocation of the cervical spine. At the time of injury, on the athletic field, there is no way to determine the presence of an unstable fracture. This requires appropriate radiographs to be taken.

There also is no way of differentiating between a fully recoverable and a permanent case of quadriplegia. If the patient is fully conscious, a cervical fracture or cervical cord injury is usually accompanied by rigid cervical muscle spasm and pain that immediately alerts the athlete and physician to the presence of such an injury. It is the unconscious athlete, unable to state that the neck hurts and whose neck muscles are not in protective spasm, who is susceptible to potential cord severance if one does not always think of the possibility of an unstable cervical spine fracture.

With an unconscious or obviously neck-injured athlete, it is imperative that no neck manipulation be carried out on the field. Definitive treatment must await appropriate radiographs at a medical facility, to which the athlete must be transported with the head and neck immobilized. There a detailed neurologic examination is carried out including motor, sensory, or reflex abnormalities, anal sphincter tone, and sensation of the perineal and sacral areas.

If the neurologic examination is normal, the next step is a lateral cervical spine radiograph. If this is also normal, a complete cervical spine series of anterior, posterior, lateral, oblique, and flexion-extension views should be obtained. This last step is important, because up to 20% of unstable cervical spine injuries may be missed when the cross table lateral cervical spine radiograph is used alone (21). It is also important to remember that in the adolescent, displacement of the second cervical vertebra over the third occurs because of the hypermobility of those segments. Failure to recognize this normal of 1 to 2 mm of subluxation variation may lead to unnecessary treatment of this pseudosubluxation.

When spinal cord injury is documented on the neurologic examination, a lateral cervical spine radiograph is taken on the still neck-immobilized patient. In this instance, oblique and flexion-extension views are not taken for fear of further injuring the spinal cord. Instead, one proceeds to a CT of the cervical spine to further define the extent of the trauma and presence of spinal cord compression by bone, disc, or hematoma. A contrast positive cervical CT is often more sensitive in showing spinal cord compression. In those tertiary institutions with a magnetic resonance scanner, this modality may be used to further define especially intraspinal pathology.

Stingers

Stingers or *burners* are colloquial terms used by athletes and trainers to describe a set of symptoms that involve pain, burning, or tingling down an arm occasionally accompanied by localized weakness. Typically, these symptoms abate within seconds or minutes, rarely persisting for days or longer. It has been estimated that a stinger will occur at least once during the career of over 50% of athletes (22).

There are two typical mechanisms by which stingers may occur—traction on the brachial plexus, or nerve root impingement within the cervical neural foramen. The majority of high-school-level injuries are of the brachial plexus type, whereas most at the college level and virtually all in the professional ranks result from a pinch phenomenon within the neural foramen.

The brachial plexus stinger commonly involves a forceful blow to the head from the side. However, it can also result from head extension or shoulder depression while the head and neck are fixed. Nerve root impingement usually occurs when the athlete's head is driven toward the shoulder pad. The dorsal spinal nerve root ganglion, which lies close to the posterior intervertebral facet joints, is pinched when the neural foramen is compressed.

With either type of stinger, the athlete experiences a shock-like sensation of pain and numbness radiating into the arm and hand. The symptoms are typically purely sensory in nature and most commonly involve the C5 and C6 dermatomes. On occasion, weakness may also be present. The most common muscles involved include the deltoid, biceps, supraspinatus, and infraspinatus.

Stingers are always unilateral and virtually never involve the lower extremities. Thus, if symptoms are bilateral or involve the legs, the burning hands syndrome with all its implications must be considered.

If there is no neck pain or limitation of neck movement, and if all motor and sensory symptoms clear within seconds to minutes, the athlete may safely return to competition. This is especially true if the athlete has previously experienced similar symptoms. If there are any residual symptoms or complaints of neck pain, return should be deferred pending further workup.

On rare occasions, a stinger may result in prolonged sensory complaints or weakness. In such a situation, an MRI of the cervical spine should be considered to look for a herniated disc or other compressive pathology. If symptoms persist for more than 2 weeks, electromyography should allow for an accurate assessment of the degree and extent of injury.

Some athletes seem predisposed to develop a series of recurrent stingers. It has been suggested that repeated stinger injuries over many years may lead to a proximal arm weakness and constant pain. Thus, if an athlete suffers two or more stingers, particularly in rapid succession, consideration should be given to the use of high shoulder pads supplemented by a soft cervical roll that should limit lateral neck flexion and extension. Examining and possibly changing the athlete's blocking and tackling techniques or changing the player's position may also be helpful in preventing recurrences. If despite these interventions the stingers repeatedly recur, the athlete may need to stop participating in contact sports.

Transient Quadriplegia

If a player displays transient quadriplegia or bilateral neurologic symptoms after taking a hit in a contact sport, there may be spinal cord compromise. In some athletes, spinal stenosis may be a contributing factor. Though radiographic bone measurements can suggest that the problem may be present, physicians are cautioned against making the diagnosis of spinal stenosis with this technique alone. Instead, diagnostic technologies that view the spinal cord itself—magnetic resonance imaging (MRI), contrast positive computed tomography (CT), or myelography—should be employed. These imaging methods can determine if the spinal cord has a normal functional reserve: the space largely filled with a protective cushion of cerebrospinal fluid between the cord and the spinal canal's interior walls lined by bone, disk, and ligament (see Figures 1.5a and 1.5b). In addition, these techniques also determine whether the nerve tissue is deformed

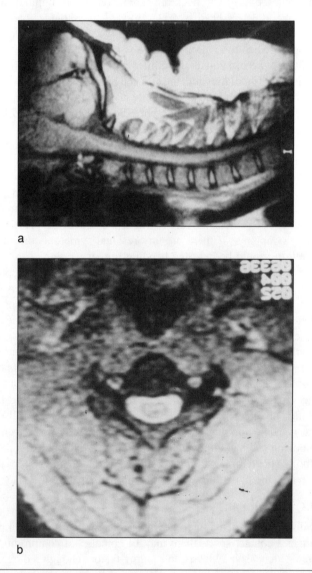

a

b

Figure 1.5 (a) Sagittal MRI. Note wide column of CSF around the spinal cord. (b) Coronal contrast positive CT showing wide column of CSF around the spinal cord.

by an abnormality such as disc protrusion, bony osteophyte, or posterior buckling of the ligamentum flavum (see Figure 1.6).

Controversy persists as to whether cervical stenosis increases the risk of spinal cord injury. I believe very strongly that those who have had spinal cord symptoms from sport-related injuries and are shown to have true spinal stenosis on MRI should not be allowed to return to contact sports.

Though there is no hard data to back up that recommendation, a body of literature in sports medicine, neurology, and radiology indicates that spinal stenosis predisposes a patient to spinal cord injury (23-29). Matsuura and his group (29), for example, compared the spinal dimensions of 100 controls with those of 42 patients who had spinal cord injuries. They found that the control group had significantly larger sagittal spinal canal diameters than did the patients who had spinal cord injuries. Furthermore, the NCCSIR has seen no instance of complete neurologic recovery in spinal stenotic athletes with fracture dislocation of the cervical spine, while there are a number of such complete recoveries in athletes with normal size spinal canals. There are also several instances of permanent quadriplegia in athletes with tight spinal stenosis without fracture or

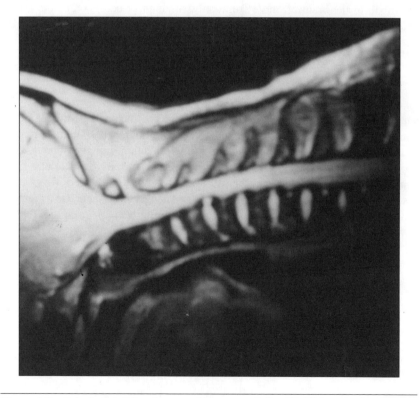

Figure 1.6 Spinal cord deformity caused by ruptured disc C3-C4 into an already functionally spinal stenotic canal. Note no CSF around the cord.

demonstrated instability. For these reasons, we are adamant that, following spinal cord symptoms, athletes exhibiting "functional spinal stenosis" should no longer participate in contact collision sports.

Increased attention soon may be focused on this question, however, as several professional football teams now require detailed investigations of the cervical and lumbar spine (some including MRIs) as a prerequisite to the draft process. Presently, there are no good guidelines to help the physician manage an athlete with a narrow asymptomatic cervical spinal canal. When such an abnormality is encountered, management must be individualized according to the patient's symptoms, the degree of canal stenosis, and the perceived risk of permanent neurologic injury.

Vascular Injury

A final uncommon but very serious neck injury involves the carotid arteries. By either extremes of lateral flexion or extension or a forceful blow by a relatively fixed, narrow object (such as a stiffened forearm or a cross-country ski tip impaling one's neck in a forward fall), the inner layer (intima) of the carotid artery may be torn. This can lead to clot formation at the site of injury, resulting in emboli to the brain or, more commonly, a complete occlusion of the artery, causing a major stroke. Especially with a fracture dislocation, injury to the vertebral artery may occur, leading to a brainstem stroke.

Conclusion

Careful study of the pathomechanics and epidemiology of sport-related spine injuries brings to light many common features. The incidence increases as the sport becomes increasingly violent and aggressive. Improperly conditioned neck muscles and lack of knowledge of the proper techniques of the sport put the athlete who sustains a blow to the head at significant risk for head and spine injury. Improper helmet fit and the use of the head as an offensive weapon are also common factors. While recognition of these dangers has resulted in a dramatic reduction in catastrophic athletic spine injury, the athlete remains at risk for less severe head and spine injuries.

References

1. Tator CH, Edmonds JE: National survey of spinal injuries in hockey players. *Can Med Assoc.* 1984;130:875.
2. Torg JS: Epidemiology, pathomechanics, and prevention of athletic injuries to the cervical spine. *Med Sci Sports Exerc.* 1985;17:295.
3. Committee on Head Injury Nomenclature of the Congress of Neurological Surgeons: Glossary of head injury including some definitions of injury to the cervical spine. *Clin Neurosurg.* 1966;12:386.
4. Maroon JC, Steele PB, Berlin R: Football head and neck injuries: an update. *Clin Neurosurg.* 1980;27:414.

 5. Jennet B: Late effects of head injuries. In: Critchley M, O'Leary JL, Jennet B (eds): *Scientific Foundations of Neurology.* Philadelphia: FA Davis Co; 1971:441.
 6. Cantu RC: Guidelines for return to contact sports after a cerebral concussion. *Phys Sports Med.* 1987;14:76-79.
 7. Yarnell PR, Lynch S: The "ding" amnestic states in football trauma. *Neurology.* 1983;23:196.
 8. Meggyesy D: *Out of their league.* Berkeley, CA: Ramparts; 1970:125.
 9. Hugenholtz H, Richard MT: Return to athletic competition following concussion. *Can Med Assoc J.* 1982;127:827.
10. Lindsay KW, McLatchie G, Jennet B: Serious head injury in sport. *Br Med J.* 1980;281:789.
11. Murphey F, Simmons JC: Initial management of athletic injuries to the head and neck. *Am J Surg.* 1959;98:379-383.
12. Guthkelch AN: Posttraumatic amnesia, postconcussional symptoms and accident neurosis. *Eur Neurol.* 1980;19:91-102.
13. Gruber R, Bubl R, Fruttiger V: Anticonvulsant therapy after juvenile craniocerebral injuries: a retrospective evaluation. *Z Kinderchir.* 1985;40:199-202.
14. Blahd WH Jr, Iserson KV, Bjelland JC: Efficiency of the posttraumatic cross table lateral view of the cervical spine. *J Emerg Med.* 1985;2:243-249.
15. Cantu RC: *Health maintenance through physical conditioning.* Littleton, MA: Wright-PSG Publishing Inc.; 1981.
16. Cantu RC: *The exercising adult.* 2nd ed. New York: MacMillan; 1987.
17. Fekete JF: Severe brain injury and death following minor hockey accidents. *Can Med Assoc J.* 1986;99:1234-1239.
18. Saunders RL, Harbaugh RE: The second impact in catastrophic contact sports head trauma. *JAMA.* 1984;252(4):538-539.
19. Schneider RC: *Head and neck injuries in football: mechanisms, treatment and prevention.* Baltimore: Williams & Wilkins; 1973.
20. Kelley JP, Nichols JS, Filley CM, et al: Concussion in sports: guidelines for the prevention of catastrophic outcome. *JAMA.* 1991;266(20):2867-2869.
21. Herzog RJ, Wiens JJ, Dillingham MF, et al: Normal cervical spine morphometry and cervical spinal stenosis in asymptomatic professional football players: plain film radiography, multiplanar computed tomography, and magnetic resonance imaging. *Spine.* 1991;16(6 suppl):S178-S186.
22. Feldick HG, Albright JP: Football survey reveals "missed" neck injuries. *Phys Sportsmed.* 1976;4:77-81.
23. Wolfe BS, Khilnani M, Malis L: The sagittal diameter of the bony cervical spinal canal and its significance in cervical spondylosis. *J Mt Sinai Hosp.* 1956;23:283-292.
24. Alexander MD, Davis CH, Field CH: Hyperextension injuries of the cervical spine. *Arch Neurol & Psychiat.* 1958;79:146-150.
25. Eismont FJ, Clifford S, Goldberg M, et al: Cervical sagittal spinal canal size in spine injury. *Spine.* 1984;9(7):663-666.
26. Penning L: Some aspects of plain radiography of the cervical spine in chronic myelopathy. *Neurology* (Minneapolis). 1962;12:513-519.

27. Mayfield FH: Neurosurgical aspects of cervical trauma. In: *Clinical Neurosurgery.* Baltimore: Williams & Wilkins; 1955: vol 2.
28. Nugent GR: Clinicopathologic correlations in cervical spondylosis. *Neurology.* 1959;9:273-281.
29. Matsuura P, Waters RL, Atkins RH, et al: Comparison of computerized tomography parameters of the cervical spine in normal control subjects and spinal cord-injured patients. *J Bone Joint Surg (AM).* 1989;71(2):183-188.

Chapter 2

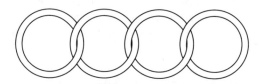

Sudden Death in Athletes

The sudden death of athletes, such as the recent highly publicized, tragic deaths of Hank Gathers (1) and Reggie Lewis (2), causes widespread public concern and questions (3). Publication by the National Center for Catastrophic Sports Injury Research (NCCSIR) of information about the frequency and causes of fatalities has resulted in improvements in equipment and changes in rules and coaching techniques in high school and college football. These improvements and changes have been associated with a subsequent reduction in catastrophic injuries (4). An increased awareness and understanding of the problem of indirect catastrophic injuries, or nontraumatic sports deaths, likewise should lead to a reduction in their occurrence.

From July 1983 through June 1993, the NCCSIR at the University of North Carolina, Chapel Hill (UNC-CH), received information regarding the occurrence of nontraumatic deaths in 160 high school and college athletes. Of these non-traumatic deaths, adequate information to classify by cause of death was obtained in 136 cases, through either autopsy data (128); coroner or medical examiner reports (3); death certificates (3); or attending physician reports (2). The information received on these 136 athletes was reviewed by a cardiovascular pathologist and a cardiologist, with additional consultations in some cases from the pathologist who had performed the autopsy, physicians involved in the athlete's care, or other medical specialists in order to establish the cause of each athlete's death.

Athletic participation data were obtained from the primary organizations concerned with high school and college athletics in the US: the National Federation of State High School Associations (NFSHSA), the National Collegiate Athletic Association (NCAA), the National Association of Intercollegiate Athletics (NAIA), the National Junior College Athletic Association (NJCAA), and the Community College League of California. These participation figures were used to calculate estimated rates of nontraumatic (indirect) death for high school and college athletes and for specific sports.

Adjustment for the participation of athletes in multiple sports each year was necessary to obtain an estimate of the total number of athletes participating at the high school and college levels. The sums of the participation figures for each sport were divided by an estimate of the average number of sports in which each high school and college athlete participated, 1.9 for high school athletes and 1.2 for college (NCAA, NAIA, NJCAA, and California Community College) athletes. Calculation of estimated rates of death in male and female high school and college sports over the 10-year study period were made using the participation figures.

Frequencies of Indirect (Nontraumatic) Deaths

For the 10-year period of July 1, 1983, through June 30, 1993, reports of 160 indirect (nontraumatic) fatalities (146 males, mean age 16.9 ± 2.0 years [13-24 years range of ages] and 14 females, mean age 16.2 ± 2.4 years [14-22 years]) in organized high school and college athletic activities were obtained. Thus the annual frequency of indirect deaths was 16 per year. These nontraumatic fatalities occurred in 126 high school athletes (115 males and 11 females), and 34 college athletes (31 males and 3 females).

The number and estimated rates of these deaths in male and female high school and college athletes are shown in Tables 2.1 and 2.2. The estimated rate of nontraumatic sports deaths in male high school and college athletes was compared with rates in female high school and college athletes, and found to be more than five times higher in males (7.47 vs. 1.33 per million athletes per year).

Table 2.1   Nontraumatic Sports Deaths in Male High School and College Athletes, July 1983-June 1993

		Total deaths	Estimated athletes participating*	Estimated death rates per million athletes per year
Fall sports				
Cross country	High school	3	1,552,413	1.93
	College	1	138,873	7.20
Field hockey	High school	0	290	0
	College	0	0	—
Football	High school	53	9,449,220	5.61
	College	14	690,219	20.28
Soccer	High school	6	2,108,958	2.85
	College	1	246,085	4.06
Water polo	High school	0	92,055	0
	College	1	16,175	61.82

		Total deaths	Estimated athletes participating*	Estimated death rates per million athletes per year
Winter sports				
Basketball	High school	28	5,112,448	5.48
	College	9	259,364	34.70
Gymnastics	High school	0	50,286	0
	College	0	8,007	0
Ice hockey	High school	1	229,655	4.35
	College	1	43,823	22.82
Swimming	High school	0	832,919	0
	College	1	98,797	10.12
Volleyball	High school	0	140,384	0
	College	0	9,747	0
Wrestling	High school	9	2,397,129	3.75
	College	0	102,388	0
Spring sports				
Baseball	High school	5	4,107,505	1.22
	College	2	389,339	5.14
Golf	High school	0	1,196,635	0
	College	0	112,722	0
Lacrosse	High school	0	180,393	0
	College	1	54,478	18.36
Tennis	High school	1	1,336,764	0.75
	College	0	123,737	0
Track	High school	9	4,296,343	2.09
	College	1	272,263	3.67
Total	High school	115	33,083,397 ÷ 1.9[†]	
			17,412,314	6.60
	College	31	2,566,017 ÷ 1.2[†]	
			2,138,348	14.50
	High school and college	146	19,550,662	7.47

*Athletes counted once for every year of participation, and for each sport in which they participated.

[†]Estimation of the total number of athletes participating requires division by estimated number of sports participated in by athletes per year (1.9 for high school athletes and 1.2 for college athletes). This estimation is then used to calculate the total estimated death rates for the high school, college, and combined high school and college groups.

Table 2.2   Nontraumatic Sports Deaths in Female High School and College Athletes, July 1983-June 1993

		Total deaths	Estimated athletes participating*	Estimated death rates per million athletes per year
Fall sports				
Cross country	High school	1	1,023,646	0.98
	College	0	105,953	0
Field hockey	High school	0	491,274	0
	College	0	51,991	0
Football	High school	0	844	0
	College	0	0	—
Soccer	High school	1	1,052,873	0.95
	College	1	84,530	11.83
Water polo	High school	0	9,006	0
	College	0	0	—
Winter sports				
Basketball	High school	4	3,907,849	1.02
	College	1	213,010	4.69
Gymnastics	High school	0	288,506	0
	College	0	17,043	0
Ice hockey	High school	0	698	0
	College	0	0	—
Swimming	High school	3	852,480	3.52
	College	0	95,277	0
Volleyball	High school	0	2,884,819	0
	College	0	188,317	0
Wrestling	High school	0	1,494	0
	College	0	0	—
Spring sports				
Golf	High school	0	323,767	0
	College	0	12,547	0
Lacrosse	High school	0	87,167	0
	College	0	29,466	0
Softball	High school	0	2,500,642	0
	College	0	199,629	0
Tennis	High school	0	1,264,627	0
	College	1	108,913	9.18
Track	High school	2	3,312,021	0.60
	College	0	175,321	0

		Total deaths	Estimated athletes participating*	Estimated death rates per million athletes per year
Total	High school	11	18,001,713	
			$\div\ 1.9^{\dagger}$	
			9,474,586	1.16
	College	3	1,281,997	
			$\div\ 1.2^{\dagger}$	
			1,068,331	2.81
	High school and college	14	10,542,917	1.33

*Athletes counted once for every year of participation, and for each sport in which they participated.

†Estimation of the total number of athletes participating requires division by estimated number of sports participated in by athletes per year (1.9 for high school athletes and 1.2 for college athletes). This estimation is then used to calculate the total estimated death rates for the high school, college, and combined high school and college groups.

This disparity is highly significant ($p < 0.0001$), and, although our study did not address male athletes' higher rates of death, they may involve

- participation at higher levels of intensity among males;
- more denial or lack of attention to warning symptoms among males;
- the generally larger cardiac size in males compared with females (5-7) in combination with other pathological conditions; and
- greater frequency of certain conditions in males (e.g., exertional hyperthermia and rhabdomyolysis) related to their generally larger body size and skeletal muscle mass.

The estimated rate of nontraumatic sports deaths was more than two times greater in male college athletes than in male high school athletes (14.50 vs. 6.60 per million athletes per year).

This disparity is also highly significant ($p < 0.0001$). Its cause(s) are unclear, but certainly merit further study. Although the estimated rate of nontraumatic sports death was similarly two times higher in female college athletes than in female high school athletes (2.81 vs. 1.16 per million per year), the number of deaths and the total sample were too small to carry out a valid test.

With regard to nontraumatic deaths in specific sports over the 10-year period, the highest number of male deaths were in high school football (53), high school basketball (28), and college football (14). For female athletes, more than one death was reported only in high school basketball (4), high school swimming (3), and high school track (2). Comparison of estimated rates of nontraumatic death in specific sports was possible only for college football because of the low number of deaths and small total sample in the other sports. The estimated rate of nontraumatic sports death was greater in male college football players compared with all other male college athletes (20.28 vs. 11.74 per million athletes per year), but was not statistically significant (p = 0.13).

Among the 160 athletes with nontraumatic sports deaths, the cause of death could be established in 136 cases. Autopsy reports were unavailable, primarily for legal reasons, in 14 cases, and autopsy was not performed in 10. Four athletes in the latter group were hospitalized from 1 to 30 days prior to death, with their cause of death established by clinical information (not available) rather than autopsy. Although these athletes, nine males and one female, did not differ significantly in general characteristics or circumstances of death from the athletes in whom cause of death could be established, they were not included in the evaluation of clinical characteristics (Table 2.3) or causes of death (Table 2.4).

The cohort of the 136 high school and college athletes in whom adequate information regarding cause of death was obtained was evaluated in both clinical (Table 2.3) and pathological (Tables 2.4-2.5) manners. Of these 136 athletes, 78 (57%) were Caucasian, 52 (38%) were African American, 3 (2%) were Hispanic, 1 (1%) was Asian, 1 (1%) was Puerto Rican, and 1 (1%) was Native American. This racial information is presented for descriptive purposes, but as no data are available regarding the racial distribution of all high school and college athletes, risk within racial groups can not be addressed.

The athletes' deaths were more frequently practice related (83) than competition related (53). However, given that practice participation times were probably 5 to 10 times greater than time spent in competition, the competition-related collapses would be proportionally increased. The fact that practice-related collapses were not 5 to 10 times more frequent probably reflects the greater intensity of activity and greater emotional stress accompanying competition.

Table 2.3 Characteristics of 136 High School and College Athletes Experiencing Nontraumatic Sports Death, July 1983-June 1993

Characteristic	Total	Male	Female
Number of athletes	136	124	12
Race—no. (%)			
Caucasian	78 (57.4%)	69 (55.6%)	9 (75%)
African American	52 (38%)	49 (39.5%)	3 (25%)
Hispanic	3 (2.2%)	3 (2.4%)	0
Asian	1 (0.7%)	1 (0.8%)	0
Puerto Rican	1 (0.7%)	1 (0.8%)	0
Native American	1 (0.7%)	1 (0.8%)	0
Activity at time of collapse—no. (%)			
Practice	83 (61%)		
Competition	53 (39%)		

Table 2.4   Causes of Nontraumatic Sports Deaths in 136 High School and College Athletes, July 1983-June 1993

Nontraumatic sports deaths	Total 136	Male 124	Female 12
Athletes with cardiovascular conditions	100*†	92*†	8
Hypertrophic cardiomyopathy	51‡§	50‡§	1
Probable hypertrophic cardiomyopathy	5	5	0
Coronary artery anomaly	16*‡	14*‡	2
Myocarditis	7‖	7‖	0
Aortic stenosis	6	6	0
Dilated cardiomyopathy	5	5	0
Atherosclerotic coronary artery disease	3	2	1
Aortic rupture	2	2	0
Cardiomyopathy—nonspecific	2‖	2‖	0
Tunnel subaortic stenosis	2#	2#	0
Coronary artery aneurysm	1	0	1
Mitral valve prolapse	1	1	0
Right ventricular cardiomyopathy	1	0	1
Ruptured cerebellar arteriovenous malformation	1	0	1
Subarachnoid hemorrhage	1	0	1
Wolff-Parkinson-White syndrome	1§	1§	0
Athletes with noncardiovascular conditions	30*	27*	3
Hyperthermia	13	12	1
Rhabdomyolysis and sickle cell trait	7*	6*	1
Status asthmaticus	4	3	1
Electrocution due to lightning	3	3	0
Arnold-Chiari II malformation	1	1	0
Aspiration-blood-GI bleed	1	1	0
Exercise-induced anaphylaxis	1	1	0
Athletes with cause of death undetermined	7	6	1

*1 male athlete had a cardiovascular condition (coronary artery anomaly) and a noncardiovascular condition (rhabdomyolysis and sickle cell trait).

†5 male athletes had multiple cardiovascular conditions.

‡3 male athletes had hypertrophic cardiomyopathy and a coronary artery anomaly.

§1 male athlete had hypertrophic cardiomyopathy and Wolff-Parkinson-White syndrome.

‖1 male athlete had myocarditis and a nonspecific cardiomyopathy.

#1 male athlete had hypoplasia of the aortic arch associated with tunnel subaortic stenosis.

Causes of Indirect (Nontraumatic) Deaths

The causes of indirect (nontraumatic) sports deaths in these 136 high school and college athletes are shown in Table 2.4. Cardiovascular conditions were found

Table 2.5   Coronary Artery Anomalies in 16 High School and College Athletes Experiencing Nontraumatic Sports Death

	Athletes
Anomalous origin of LCA from right sinus of Valsalva	4
Intramural LAD	4*‡
Anomalous origin of LCA from PA	2
Anomalous origin of RCA from left sinus of Valsalva	2‡
Congenital hypoplasia RCA	2
Anomalous inferior origin of LCA with ostial ridge	1
Ostial ridge at origin of LCA	1
Total	16

LAD = left anterior descending coronary artery.

LCA = left coronary artery.

PA = pulmonary artery.

RCA = right coronary artery.

*2 athletes had this coronary artery anomaly in combination with hypertrophic cardiomyopathy.

†1 athlete had this coronary artery anomaly and exertional rhabdomyolysis and sickle cell trait.

‡1 athlete had this coronary artery anomaly in combination with hypertrophic cardiomyopathy.

in 100 athletes, 92 males and 8 females. Five of these male athletes were found to have multiple cardiovascular disorders.

Hypertrophic cardiomyopathy was the most frequent cause of nontraumatic death, occurring in 51 of the 136 athletes. As has previously been reported, this condition is the most frequently found disorder among young athletes dying suddenly (8, 9). It has also been reported (10, 11) as a cause of sudden death in athletes over 30 years of age, but at a much lower incidence than in studies of younger athletes.

In this condition, the left ventricle is hypertrophied but not dilated. This hypertrophy has an underlying genetic basis occurring in the absence of a cardiac or systemic condition that could produce ventricular hypertrophy, such as aortic stenosis or systemic hypertension. The intraventricular septal thickness is typically 15 mm or greater, with left ventricular free wall thickness either normal or also increased.

Two additional pathologic features that likely contribute to the potential for fatal arrhythmias are typically present. These are myocardial cellular disarray and abnormally thickened intramural coronary arteries with narrow lumens.

Of the 51 athletes with hypertrophic cardiomyopathy, 50 (98%) were males and only 1 (2%) was a female. The reasons for this finding are likely multiple. As with nontraumatic sports deaths in general, the factors of higher male participation frequency, intensity of activity, and denial or lack of attention to prodromal symptoms may certainly be operative. Additionally, males with hypertrophic cardiomyopathy are more likely to have greater cardiac weights than females, possibly thereby increasing the risk of sudden death.

Additional pathological findings or clinical histories were considered to be significant and possibly contributory to death in four cases: coronary artery anomalies in three athletes, and a history of Wolff-Parkinson-White syndrome in one.

Five athletes, all males, were classified as having probable hypertrophic cardiomyopathy. These athletes had significant cardiac hypertrophy although not to the extent required in our classification of hypertrophic cardiomyopathy. With respect to clinical histories, these five athletes were not significantly different from those with hypertrophic cardiomyopathy. They are therefore considered along with those with hypertrophic cardiomyopathy with regard to clinical characteristics.

Thirty-three (59%) of these 56 athletes were Caucasian, 20 (36%) were African American, 1 (2%) was Native American, 1 (2%) was Asian, and 1 (2%) was Puerto Rican. The racial distribution of athletes with hypertrophic cardiomyopathy thus paralleled that of all the athletes taken together (Table 2.3). None of these athletes was known to have a positive family history for hypertrophic cardiomyopathy.

Coronary artery anomalies, occurring in 16 athletes, 14 males and 2 females (Table 2.5), represented the second most commonly found pathological condition causing indirect deaths in our study population. These have been found in other series of exertional sudden deaths (8, 9, 12, 13). In these conditions, there is an anomalous coronary artery origin or course, including an intramural coronary artery. These anomalies may result in myocardial ischemia and fatal arrhythmias during exercise. Possible mechanisms include coronary artery constriction (at the coronary orifice or along its arterial course) and anatomic inadequacy (coronary artery hypoplasia).

An anomalous origin of the left coronary artery (LCA) from the right sinus of Valsalva, a well-recognized cause of exercise-related sudden death (8, 14), was present in four cases, as was an intramural left anterior descending (LAD) coronary artery. In only one of the four athletes with an intramural LAD was it the only pathologic abnormality. Two athletes with an intramural LAD coronary artery also had hypertrophic cardiomyopathy, and one also had exertional rhabdomyolysis and sickle cell trait. This latter athlete's collapse and clinical course suggested that both the intramural LAD and the rhabdomyolysis and related sickle cell trait were primary factors in his death.

Although reported and generally accepted as a cause of exercise-related sudden death (15, 16), the significance of intramural LAD coronary arteries has been questioned (17), primarily because of their frequent occurrence (27%) in general autopsies series (15). Other coronary artery anomalies found included: anomalous origin of the left coronary artery (LCA) from the pulmonary artery (two cases); anomalous origin of the right coronary artery (RCA) from the left sinus of Valsalva (two cases); congenital hypoplasia of the right coronary artery (RCA) (two cases); and single cases of an ostial ridge at the origin of the LCA, and an anomalous inferior origin of the LCA with a slit-like ostium.

The two cases of anomalous origin of the left coronary artery from the pulmonary artery are very noteworthy. This condition was found in athletes competing in water polo and wrestling. Reports of this condition in medical literature usually emphasize the presentation of this anomaly in infants with a myocardial infarction and congestive heart failure (18), certainly different from the presentation of these two athletes who were both competing in strenuous athletic endeavors.

This anomaly was found in both athletes in conjunction with myocardial fibrosis. The fatal arrhythmias in these two athletes probably resulted from inadequate coronary flow of oxygenated blood in the presence of myocardial fibrosis.

Myocarditis, characterized pathologically by the presence of myocardial inflammation and necrosis, is often difficult to establish clinically. Previously recognized to be a cause of exercise-related sudden death (19-21), it was found to be responsible for seven deaths. Active, along with healed, myocarditis with resultant myocardial fibrosis is considered to be an abnormal myocardial substrate which may result in life-threatening arrhythmias (22). These deaths are the basis for medical recommendations that athletes with significant viral illness not compete until the illness has resolved.

While myocarditis is generally considered to be of infectious, usually viral, origin, it should be remembered that cocaine abuse may also lead to myocardial inflammation (23, 24). It therefore should be considered in any case of unexplained myocarditis. Our study, confined to deaths related to high school- or college-sponsored athletic activity, did not find any deaths related to drug abuse.

This absence is especially noteworthy given media reports of multiple drug-related sudden deaths among professional and former professional athletes in recent years (including Len Bias, Don Rogers, David Croudip, and Dave Waymer). We did not include these deaths in our study because they were not related to sport activities and they were not in our population study group (high school and college athletes).

Congenital aortic valvular stenosis was considered the cause of death in six athletes, and tunnel subaortic stenosis with a fibrous band inferior to the aortic valve in two. Tunnel subaortic stenosis, which accounts for 8% to 10% of all cases of congenital aortic stenosis (25), has been reported as a cause of sudden, though not sports, death (26). As it pathophysiologically resembles congenital aortic stenosis, it certainly must be recognized as a potentially lethal abnormality. These two conditions would be expected to have easily detectable heart murmurs, facilitating proper diagnosis and athletic restriction.

Cardiomyopathies other than hypertrophic cardiomyopathy [dilated (5), nonspecific (2), and right ventricular (1)] were found infrequently in these athletes, as has been reported in other series (8, 9, 12). The dilated cardiomyopathies were characterized grossly by biventricular dilation and fibrosis and microscopically by interstitial fibrosis and focal hypertrophy of myocardial cells.

Right ventricular cardiomyopathy has been reported as a frequent cause of sudden death by only one group, whose subjects were gathered from a single region of northern Italy (27). This finding lends strength to the concept of a genetic basis for this cardiomyopathy. Interestingly, the paternal ancestors of the only victim of right ventricular cardiomyopathy in our study were from northern Italy.

Acquired coronary artery disease was found in four athletes, two males and two females. The two males and one female were found to have significant atherosclerotic coronary artery disease, each with areas of myocardial scarring. The other female was found to have an aneurysm of her left anterior descending coronary artery (possibly secondary to Kawasaki's disease) with partial thrombosis.

Aortic disease was found in three athletes, all males. Two had a ruptured aortic aneurysm, including one with Marfan syndrome, which has previously been described as a cause of sudden death in athletes (8, 28). A third athlete had a congenital hypoplasia of the aorta (approximately half the size of his pulmonary artery) with secondary left ventricular hypertrophy.

Mitral valve prolapse with myxomatous change of the mitral valve leaflets was identified as the cause of death in one athlete. This condition has also been found on postmortem examination of exercising sudden death victims (9, 29). However, as it is also found frequently in the general population, its role in the pathogenesis of exercise-related sudden death is unclear, though generally considered to be minor. Cerebral hemorrhage, due to a subarachnoid hemorrhage and a ruptured arteriovenous malformation, was responsible for the deaths of two female athletes.

Noncardiovascular conditions were the cause of death in 30 (22%) of the 136 athletes. It is of major significance that they are, for the most part, preventable. Especially important in this context is exertional hyperthermia. This condition was the cause of death in 13 athletes, 12 males and 1 female.

It is generally believed that a high level of awareness exists among coaches and athletic trainers regarding the potentially catastrophic effects of hyperthermia. Nevertheless, fatalities due to exertional hyperthermia have continued through the last decade. Most deaths followed collapse during football practice (11) or conditioning runs (2) during August and September, in hot, usually humid, environments. They usually occurred in large athletes who not only generate a large heat burden, but also have more difficulty in dissipating it.

Of the 11 football players, 9 were African American, 1 was Caucasian, and 1 was Hispanic. The other two athletes were both Caucasian. The football players were large athletes, including one 6-ft, 334-lb lineman, five between 260 and 296 lb and four between 200 and 230 lb. All athletes were transported to hospitals after initial collapse, with deaths occurring within a few hours in two and from 1 to 9 days later in the others. A history of prior collapse during heat was reported in only one case.

Death due to exertional rhabdomyolysis occurred in seven athletes with sickle cell trait, six male football players and one female basketball player. All were African American. Of the football players, five collapsed during the first day of conditioning drills involving timed runs. The 20-year-old female collapsed at the end of a 3-mile training run.

These deaths were unexpected, as sickle cell trait is generally viewed as being without adverse physiologic or health consequences. However, it has been reported as both a factor in cases of exertion-induced rhabdomyolysis in military recruits (30) and as a primary factor in cases of exertional rhabdomyolysis in athletes (31). Especially vulnerable appear to be those athletes with sickle cell trait who perform maximal, or "heroic," exercise in pre-season conditioning sessions, as was the case in six of the seven athletes in this study.

In consideration of this problem, the inevitable issue of screening for sickle cell trait in athletes surfaces. An athlete found to have sickle cell trait would be known to be at increased risk from overexertion, dehydration, and overheating, particularly if unaccustomed to high-intensity activity. However, screening programs would necessitate additional expense and would have to be considered for those of non-African descent, in whom the prevalence is 1 in 10,000, as well as in those of African descent, in whom the prevalence is 8%.

An alternative approach would be to

- avoid prolonged high-intensity activity in unacclimatized individuals;
- stress the avoidance of dehydration and overheating; and
- treat any occurrences of prolonged (greater than 15 min) generalized muscle cramps as medical emergencies.

Afflicted individuals should be cooled, hydrated, and immediately transported to an emergency medical facility for definitive evaluation, monitoring, and treatment.

Status asthmaticus was responsible for 4 of the 30 noncardiovascular deaths. Three were males and one was female. Autopsy findings included mucous plugging and edema of bronchi and bronchioles, smooth muscle and bronchial mucosal hyperplasia, and marked cellular inflammation. All had prior histories of bronchial asthma. These deaths due to asthma highlight the issue that exercise-induced bronchospasm may not only be a detriment to performance, but in rare instances may be life threatening.

Exercise-induced anaphylaxis occurred in a male distance runner who collapsed during a 2-mile race in cold, windy weather. Autopsy findings showed his larynx to be markedly edematous with almost complete obstruction. He was known to have had asthma since childhood and was taking oral theophylline, but had no prior history of anaphylaxis, urticaria, or angioedema.

Electrocution due to lightning occurred in three athletes. A nontraumatic central nervous system condition, an Arnold-Chiari II malformation with cerebellar tonsillar herniation, was responsible for the death of one athlete. Also, one death was attributed to asphyxia due to aspiration of blood from an esophageal tear.

In seven athletes, six males and one female, cause of death was not determined by autopsy. These deaths were most likely due to primary cardiac arrhythmias. Toxicology studies were performed in six of these cases and were negative in each.

In those cases where no pathological diagnosis was established at autopsy and cause of death was undetermined, the question of the adequacy of the autopsy arises. Conditions may have been present which carry an increased risk of exercise-related sudden death, but do not have pathological abnormalities identifiable on post-mortem examination. These would include Wolff-Parkinson-White syndrome, idiopathic long QT syndrome, and familial or primary ventricular tachycardia.

Cardiac conduction system abnormalities may also go undetected unless a detailed pathological examination is performed (32). In some cases, hypertrophic cardiomyopathy may have been present, but was not identified at autopsy. This possibility must be considered especially in view of reports of sudden deaths due to hypertrophic cardiomyopathy in the absence of cardiac hypertrophy (33, 34).

Similarly, cases of right ventricular cardiomyopathy may have been overlooked because of insufficient evaluation at the right ventricular myocardium at autopsy. It is noteworthy that cases in which the cause of death could not be determined were infrequent.

Prevention of Indirect (Nontraumatic) Deaths

These data from the largest and most comprehensive national study of nontraumatic deaths in high school and college athletes in the U.S. provide information which should assist in three important sports medicine issues:

1. Appropriate preparticipation exams
2. Eligibility recommendations for athletic participation
3. Evaluation and medical treatment of athletes

An important part of preparticipation examinations is the attempt to identify athletes with conditions which would make participation in athletics dangerous, or which require treatment prior to participation. Therefore, these examinations must be based on knowledge of the conditions which cause nontraumatic sports deaths.

Because hypertrophic cardiomyopathy is the most common cause of this tragedy, its detection requires careful consideration. Unfortunately, efforts using echocardiography on a screening basis are not considered appropriate because of their high expense and low yield (35-37).

Unfortunately, the other cardiovascular conditions placing athletes at risk for sudden death, with the exception of aortic stenosis and Marfan syndrome, are also difficult to detect, as these may have no associated symptoms or physical findings. If, however, (a) physical findings such as loud cardiac murmurs, or ones which increase in intensity with Valsalva maneuver, are present; (b) symptoms suggestive of cardiovascular abnormality such as syncope, near syncope, chest pain, or cardiac arrhythmias occur (especially with exertion); or (c) a family history of hypertrophic cardiomyopathy or unexplained premature sudden death is known, more extensive evaluations are warranted.

Conversely, the primary noncardiovascular conditions causing nontraumatic sports death (hyperthermia, exertional rhabdomyolysis) are eminently preventable, as discussed previously. Stressing to coaches that athletes will experience fewer catastrophic heat injuries and perform better if well hydrated and not overheated should persuade them to modify practice sessions when appropriate, and to use adequate hydration techniques.

Detection and proper treatment of bronchospasm prior to participation would improve physical performance in many athletes and, one hopes, prevent further fatal asthma attacks.

Recommendations regarding eligibility for competition in athletes with known cardiovascular abnormalities is an important issue which has recently been readdressed by the American College of Cardiology and the American College of Sports Medicine (38, 39). Information and insights from our study should be helpful in supplementing these recommendations.

Observation of athletes for exertional difficulties—including overheating, prolonged generalized muscular cramping, inappropriate dyspnea, lightheadedness, or chest discomfort—is critical to prevention of nontraumatic sports deaths during sporting activities. Also important is rapid response with emergency treatment to an athletic field collapse. It can never be assumed that an exercise-related collapse is a simple fainting spell due to neurally-mediated syncope or fatigue. Instead adequacy of airway, effective breathing, and circulation must be established immediately in any athlete who collapses.

Conclusion

Further study of the problem of catastrophic sports injuries, including indirect deaths, should address the reasons for increased risk in males relative to females, and in college athletes relative to high school athletes. Despite our best efforts, it is likely that nontraumatic sports deaths in high school and college athletes will continue to occur. Fortunately, the frequency of these tragedies, about 16 per year, is quite small among the approximately 3 million high school and college athletes. Awareness of the pathological conditions underlying these deaths, however, can probably lead to a reduction of their occurrence.

References

1. Maron BJ: Sudden death in young athletes: lessons from the Hank Gathers affair. *N Engl J Med.* 1993;329:55-57.
2. Van Camp SP: What can we learn from Reggie Lewis' death? *Phys Sportsmed.* 1993;21:73-97.

3. Rhoden WC: Deaths of teen-age athletes raise questions over testing. *The New York Times.* March 14, 1994;Sect A:1(col. 5).

4. Mueller FO, Cantu RC: Catastrophic injuries and fatalities in high school and college sports, fall 1982-spring 1988. *Med Sci Sports Exerc.* 1990; 22:737-741.

5. Scholz DG, Kitzman DW, Hagen PT, Ilstrup DM, Edwards WD: Age-related changes in normal human hearts during the first 10 decades of life. Part I (growth). A quantitative anatomic study of 200 specimens from subjects from birth to 19 years old. *Mayo Clin Proc.* 1988;63:126-136.

6. Kitzman DW, Scholz DG, Hagen PT, Ilstrup DM, Edwards WD: Age-related changes in normal human hearts during the first 10 decades of life. Part II (maturity). A qualitative anatomic study of 765 specimens from subjects 20 to 99 years old. *Mayo Clin Proc.* 1988;63:137-146.

7. Zeek PM: Heart weight: the weight of the normal human heart. *Arch Path.* 1942;34:820-832.

8. Maron BJ, Roberts WC, McAllister HA, Rosing DR, Epstein SE: Sudden death in young athletes. *Circulation.* 1980;62:218-229.

9. Waller BF: Exercise-related sudden death in young (age < 30 years) and older (age > 30 years) conditioned subjects. In: Wenger NK (ed): *Exercise and the Heart.* 2nd ed. Philadelphia: FA Davis; 1985:9-73.

10. Noakes TD, Rose AG, Opie LH: Hypertrophic cardiomyopathy associated with sudden death during marathon racing. *Br Heart J.* 1979;41:624-627.

11. Northcote RJ, Flannigan C, Ballantyne D: Sudden death and vigorous exercise: a study of 60 deaths associated with squash. *Br Heart J.* 1986;55: 198-203.

12. Burke AP, Farb A, Virmani R, Goodin J, Smialek JE: Sports-related and non-sports-related sudden death in young adults. *Am J Cardiol.* 1991;2:568-575.

13. Taylor AJ, Rogan KM, Virmani R: Sudden cardiac death associated with isolated congenital coronary anomalies. *J Am Coll Cardiol.* 1992;20:640-647.

14. Cheitlin MD, DeCastro CM, McAllister HA: Sudden death as a complication of anomalous left coronary origin from the anterior sinus of Valsalva: a not-so-minor congenital anomaly. *Circulation.* 1975;50:780-787.

15. Morales AR, Romanelli R, Boucek RJ: The mural left anterior descending coronary artery, strenuous exercise and sudden death. *Circulation.* 1980; 62:230-237.

16. Corrado D, Thiene G, Cocco P, Frescura C: Non-atherosclerotic coronary artery disease and sudden death in the young. *Br Heart J.* 1992;68:601-607.

17. Cheitlin MD: The intramural coronary artery: another cause of sudden death with exercise? *Circulation.* 1980;62:238-239.

18. Freidman WF: Congenital heart disease in infancy and childhood. In: Braunwald E (ed): *Heart Disease: A Textbook of Cardiovascular Medicine.* 4th ed. Philadelphia: W.B. Saunders; 1991:918-919.

19. Jokl E: Sudden death after exercise due to myocarditis. In: Jokl E, McClellan JT (eds): *Exercise and Cardiac Death. Medicine and Sport.* Basel: Karger; 1971;5:115-165.

20. Phillips M, Robinowitz M, Higgins JR, Boran KJ, Reed C, Virmani R: Sudden cardiac death in Air Force recruits: a 20-year study. *JAMA*. 1986;256:2696-2699.

21. Drory Y, Turets Y, Hiss Y, et al: Sudden unexpected death in persons < 40 years of age. *Am J Cardiol*. 1991;68:1388-1392.

22. Lecomte D, Fornes P, Fouret P, Nicholas G: Isolated myocardial fibrosis as a cause of sudden cardiac death and its possible relation to myocarditis. *J Forensic Sci*. 1993;48:617-621.

23. Isner JM, Estes NAM, Thompson PD, et al: Acute cardiac events temporally related to cocaine abuse. *New Engl J Med*. 1986;326:1438-1443.

24. Virmani R, Robinowitz M, Smialek JE, Smyth DF: Cardiovascular effects of cocaine: an autopsy study of 40 patients. *Am Heart J*. 1988;115:1068-1075.

25. Friedman WF: Congenital heart disease in infancy and childhood. In: Braunwald E (ed): *Heart disease: A Textbook of Cardiovascular Medicine*. 4th ed. Philadelphia: W.B. Saunders; 1992:925.

26. James TN, Jordan JD, Riddick L, Bargeron LM: Subaortic stenosis and sudden death. *J Thorac Cardiovasc Surg*. 1988;95:247-254.

27. Thiene G, Nava A, Corrado D, Rossi L, Penelli N: Right ventricular cardiomyopathy and sudden death in young people. *N Engl J Med*. 1988;318:126-133.

28. Demak R: Marfan syndrome: a silent killer. *Sports Illustrated*. 1986;64:30-35.

29. Virmani R, Robinowitz M, McAllister HA: Nontraumatic death in joggers: a series of 30 patients at autopsy. *Am. J. Med*. 1982;72:874-881.

30. Koppes GM, Daly JJ, Coltman CA, Butkus DE: Exertion-induced rhabdomyolysis with acute renal failure and disseminated intravascular coagulation with sickle cell trait. *Am J Med*. 1977;63:313-317.

31. Eichner ER: Sickle cell trait, heroic exercise, and fatal collapse. *Phys Sportsmed*. 1993;21:51-64.

32. James TN, Froggart P, Marshall TK: Sudden death in young athletes. *Ann Intern Med*. 1967;67:1013-1021.

33. McKenna WJ, Stewart JT, Nihoyannopoulos P, McGinty F, Davies MJ: Hypertrophic cardiomyopathy without hypertrophy: two families with myocardial disarray in the absence of increased myocardial mass. *Br Heart J*. 1990;63:287-290.

34. Maron BJ, Kragel AH, Roberts WC: Sudden death due to hypertrophic cardiomyopathy in the absence of increased left ventricular mass. *Br Heart J*. 1990;63:308-310.

35. Epstein SE, Maron BJ: Sudden death and the competitive athlete: perspectives on preparticipation screening studies. *J Am Coll Cardiol*. 1986;7:220-230.

36. Maron BJ, Bodison SA, Wesley YE, Tucker E, Gren KJ: Results of screening a large group of intercollegiate competitive athletes for cardiovascular disease. *J Am Coll Cardiol*. 1987;10:1214-1221.

37. Lewis JF, Maron BJ, Dreys JA: Preparticipation echocardiographic screening for cardiovascular disease in a large predominantly black population of collegiate athletes. *Am J Cardiol*. 1989;64:1029-1033.

38. Maron BJ, Mitchell JH: 26th Bethesda Conference: Recommendation for determining eligibility for competition in athletes with cardiovascular abnormalities. *J Am Coll Cardiol*. 1994;24:845-899.
39. Maron BJ, Mitchell JH: 26th Bethesda Conference: Recommendation for determining eligibility for competition in athletes with cardiovascular abnormalities. *Med Sci Sports Exerc*. 1994;S10:S223-S283.

Chapter 3

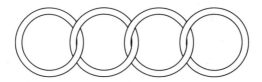

Football

Injuries in intercollegiate football date back to the very beginnings of the game (in 1869, when Princeton played Rutgers). In the late 1800s, the players wore street clothing, and football helmets were not used until 1896. Strategy played a minor role in those games, and the determining factors in winning or losing were brute force, physical conditioning, and endurance.

The 1905 football season ended in a protest against the brutality of play, and the *Chicago Tribune*'s compilation of injuries revealed 18 deaths and 159 serious injuries. In midseason, President Roosevelt met with representatives from Yale, Harvard, and Princeton, and told them that it was time to save the sport by removing every objectionable feature.

At the same time, the president of the University of California told football officials that the game must be changed or abolished, and Columbia University dropped the sport until 1915. Due to the threats to abolish football, rules were initiated in 1906 to eliminate roughness of play and the danger of injury for the player (1).

Football is one of the few sports, if not the only one, on which injury data has been collected on a national basis for many years. For this reason, this chapter will include data collected prior to 1982.

The *Annual Survey of Football Injury Research*

In 1931, the American Football Coaches Association (AFCA) initiated the *First Annual Survey of Football Fatalities* (2). Marvin A. Stevens, M.D., of Yale University directed the research until 1942, when Floyd R. Eastwood, Ph.D., of Purdue University became director. In 1965, the research came to the University of North Carolina at Chapel Hill (UNC-CH) under the direction of Carl S. Blyth, Ph.D. In 1980, Frederick O. Mueller, Ph.D., took over leadership of the project. That year, the title of the research was changed to the *Annual Survey of Football Injury Research*.

The primary purpose of the *Annual Survey of Football Injury Research* is to make the game safer for the participants. This research has been responsible for many of modern football's safety features. Among these have been rule changes—most notably the 1976 rule change that made it illegal to make contact with the head or face while blocking or tackling. In addition, there have been improvements in protective equipment and coaching techniques.

It should be noted that the 1990 report was historic in that it was the first year since the beginning of the research in 1931 that there was not a direct fatality at any level of play.

Incidence and Reduction
of Direct Football Fatalities (1960-1992)

There were 388 direct football fatalities in junior/senior high school and college football from 1960 through 1992. Junior/senior high school football was associated with 349 of these and college football with 39. It is important to point out that in 1994 1,500,000 football players were participating at the junior and senior high school level and 75,000 at the college level.

According to Table 3.1, which shows the number of fatalities for individual years from 1960 to 1992, a high number of football deaths occurred in the 1960s. In 1968, football fatalities were at an all-time high, with 26 at the junior/senior high school level and 5 at the college level for a total of 31. After 1968, there was a gradual decline in football fatalities to zero fatalities in 1990, three in 1991, and two in 1992.

Table 3.2 (page 44) illustrates that the football fatality incidence rate per 100,000 participants was less than 1 per 100,000 participants at the junior/senior high school levels and 0.00 at the college level for the years 1987 through 1992. Participation numbers changed from 1960 to 1992, and those changes are reflected in the rates. The rate per 100,000 participants for the entire period from 1960 through 1992 was 1.01 for the junior/senior high school levels and 1.64 for the college level.

Tables 3.3 and 3.4 (pages 44 and 45) show that the greatest number of fatalities at the junior/senior high school and college levels involve the head and neck. From 1960 to 1992, 85.7% of the junior/senior high school fatalities resulted from injuries to the head and neck, as did 89.6% of the college fatalities. Junior/senior high school fatalities in games outnumber those in practice by two to one, and the numbers at the college level are divided almost evenly between practice and games. Following are actual direct fatality case studies reported to the National Center for Catastrophic Sports Injury Research (NCCSIR):

Table 3.1   Fatalities: Directly Due to Football, 1960-1992

Year	High school	College	Total
1960	11	1	12
1961	10	6	16
1962	12	0	12
1963	12	2	14
1964	21	3	24
1965	20	1	21
1966	20	0	20
1967	16	3	19
1968	26	5	31
1969	18	1	19
1970	23	3	26
1971	15	3	18
1972	16	2	18
1973	7	0	7
1974	10	1	11
1975	13	1	14
1976	15	0	15
1977	8	1	9
1978	9	0	9
1979	3	1	4
1980	9	0	9
1981	5	2	7
1982	7	0	7
1983	4	0	4
1984	4	1	5
1985	4	1	5
1986	11	1	12
1987	4	0	4
1988	7	0	7
1989	4	0	4
1990	0	0	0
1991	3	0	3
1992	2	0	2
Total	349	39	388

Case Studies

A 16-year-old high school player was injured in a scrimmage game and died a day after the injury. He was playing linebacker and was struck in the chin while being blocked as he attempted to tackle the ball carrier on a goal-line stand. Autopsy reports show cause of death as a subdural hematoma.

Table 3.2   Direct Football Fatalities Rate per 100,000, 1960-1992

Year	High school	College	Year	High school	College
1960	1.78	1.53	1977	0.53	1.33
1961	1.62	9.23	1978	0.60	0.00
1962	1.94	0.00	1979	0.23	1.33
1963	1.94	3.04	1980	0.69	0.00
1964	2.23	4.56	1981	0.38	2.67
1965	2.00	1.33	1982	0.54	0.00
1966	2.00	0.00	1983	0.30	0.00
1967	1.60	4.00	1984	0.30	1.33
1968	2.60	6.60	1985	0.30	1.33
1969	1.64	1.33	1986	0.73	1.33
1970	1.92	4.00	1987	0.30	0.00
1971	1.25	4.00	1988	0.46	0.00
1972	1.33	2.67	1989	0.27	0.00
1973	0.58	0.00	1990	0.00	0.00
1974	0.83	1.33	1991	0.20	0.00
1975	1.08	1.33	1992	0.13	0.00
1976	1.00	0.00			

Participation numbers have changed over the years and these changes are reflected in the yearly rates. Since 1989, the participation numbers are 1,500,000 for senior and junior high schools and 75,000 for colleges.

Table 3.3   Direct Football Fatalities: Body Part Injured, High School, 1960-1992

Body part	Number	Percentage
Head	248	71.1
Neck	51	14.6
Brainstem	17	4.9
Heart	9	2.6
Spleen	7	2.0
Viscera	5	1.4
Kidney	2	0.6
Liver	2	0.6
Other	4	1.1
Unknown	4	1.1
Total	349	100.0

Table 3.4   Direct Football Fatalities: Body Part Injured, College, 1960-1992

Body part	Number	Percentage
Head	21	53.8
Neck	14	35.8
Viscera	1	2.6
Kidney	1	2.6
Spleen	1	2.6
Other	1	2.6
Total	39	100.0

A 17-year-old high school player was injured in a game and died 4 days after the injury. During the game, he complained to teammates of feeling dizzy. Two plays later, he ran into the quarterback on a play when he was supposed to carry the ball and collapsed on the field. He died from a subdural hematoma.

A 17-year-old high school player died 7 days after being injured in a game. He collapsed on the field after he received a hard hit while attempting to block an opponent on a first quarter kick-off. Cause of death was a subdural hematoma.

A 19-year-old college player died 5 days after being injured in a practice session. The player, a defensive tackle, received a blow to the head during a three-quarter speed drill and collapsed on the field. Cause of death was a subdural hematoma.

Head and neck football fatalities remain a concern, but the numbers have dropped dramatically. To understand the reduction that occurred after 1968, it is important to know what was happening in football in the 1960s. During this period terms like "spearing," "butt blocking and tackling," "face to the numbers," and "face to the chest" were often heard in football circles. All of the terms mentioned were associated with the techniques of blocking and tackling that coaches were teaching their players.

These tactics involved placing the face of the tackler or blocker into the chest of the opponent so that initial contact was being made with the head or face. Players were wearing full face masks and felt well protected when striking with the head or face.

Everyone associated with football was concerned with the increased number of fatalities, however, and in 1974, a National Collegiate Athletic Association (NCAA) Football Technical Committee was appointed to clarify acceptable teaching methods and techniques for blocking and tackling (3). The committee included the following members:

- Dr. Carl Blyth, University of North Carolina at Chapel Hill
- Dr. Harold Lahar, Southwest Athletic Conference
- Dr. Fred Behling, team physician at Stanford University
- Coach Wayne Harding, Temple University
- Coach Al Onofrio, University of Missouri
- Coach Eddie Robinson, Grambling University
- Coach Alex Agase, Purdue University
- James Orwig, Athletic Director, Indiana University

After considerable discussion, the committee presented recommendations concerning blocking and tackling techniques. Following is a summary of those recommendations:

1. Improper head position is the major cause of head and neck injuries. Techniques and teaching methods that require the use of the head are not recommended.
2. All coaches should stress the importance of proper head position and should explain this to the players.
3. Emphasis should be placed on having the face up with bowed neck when blocking and tackling.
4. Rules related to the malicious use of the head should be strictly enforced.

At the 1976 AFCA meeting in St. Louis, MO, the topic of head and neck injuries was discussed thoroughly (4). The Association drafted a statement for the "Football Code—Coaching Ethics" section of the NCAA Football Rule Book. The statement included the following areas:

1. The helmet shall not be used as the brunt of the contact in blocking and tackling.
2. Self-propelled mechanical apparatus (tackling dummies that were propelled by a spring loaded device) shall not be used in the teaching of blocking and tackling.
3. Players, coaches, and officials should place greater emphasis on eliminating spearing.

The gradual reduction in direct football fatalities has been a team effort by the NCAA, the AFCA, and the National Federation of State High School Associations (NFSHSA). The NCAA Football Rules Committee discussed the head and neck injury problem at their annual meeting in January 1976, and changed the rules that year to state that no player shall intentionally strike a runner with the crown or top of his helmet. The NFSHSA had already written the proposed rule changes that would make butt blocking and face tackling illegal.

In addition to the rule changes mentioned above, the National Operating Committee on Standards in Athletic Equipment (NOCSAE) established a safety standard for football helmets in 1973, and the first helmets were tested in 1974. The NOCSAE Standard was accepted by the NCAA for the 1978 football season and by the NFSHSA for the 1980 football season. It is now mandatory for all junior/senior high school and college football players to wear NOCSAE-certified helmets.

It is imperative in football head and neck injuries to gather as much information as possible concerning the football helmet being worn at the time of the injury. If a large number of the injuries are taking place with players wearing a particular brand or model helmet, notice can be made to the manufacturer and to schools and colleges that a particular helmet has been associated with a high injury rate.

Indirect Football Fatalities (1960-1992)

In many cases, fatal injuries cannot be directly related to football, and therefore were listed as indirect fatalities for the purpose of this research. Included in this category are heat stroke deaths, heart-related deaths, and any injuries recorded by the medical authorities as natural deaths. For the 33 years from 1960 through 1992 (Table 3.5, page 48), there were 215 indirect deaths associated with junior/senior high school football and 56 with college football.

The highest number during this period occurred in 1965, with 19 indirect deaths—14 in junior/senior high school and 5 in college. The numbers have been reduced since 1965, but have averaged 6.8 per year since 1980. In 1992, there were 10 indirect deaths.

Table 3.6 (page 49) shows the rates for indirect fatalities for both high school and college football. The rate for the period from 1960 through 1992 was 0.61 for the high school level and 2.30 for the college level.

Table 3.7 (page 49) shows the types of injuries associated with high school indirect football fatalities. Heart-related injuries were the leading cause, accounting for 97 deaths or 45.1% of the indirect fatalities. Heat stroke deaths are ranked second, accounting for 64 deaths or 29.8% of the total. Approximately 75% of the indirect football fatalities at the high school level were associated with heart attacks and heat stroke. All other injury types listed in Table 3.7 account for the remaining 25% of the indirect deaths. The cause of 7.9% were unknown.

The majority of the college indirect fatalities, 60.7%, were also associated with heart-related injuries and heat stroke (Table 3.8, page 50). Medical complications associated with a football injury were involved in 10.7% of the indirect fatalities. Heart-related case studies are as follows:

Case Studies

A 16-year-old high school player collapsed during a game and died 1 hr later in the hospital. The coroner listed the cause of death as idiopathic cardiomyopathy.

A 13-year-old junior high school player collapsed following practice in preseason. There was no autopsy, and the physician presumed that the death was heart related.

Table 3.5   Fatalities: Indirectly Due to Football, 1960-1992

Year	High school	College	Total
1960	2	2	4
1961	11	0	11
1962	4	2	6
1963	4	2	6
1964	12	1	13
1965	14	5	19
1966	6	2	8
1967	4	1	5
1968	8	2	10
1969	8	3	11
1970	12	2	14
1971	7	2	9
1972	10	1	11
1973	5	3	8
1974	5	3	8
1975	3	3	6
1976	7	2	9
1977	6	0	6
1978	8	1	9
1979	8	1	9
1980	4	0	4
1981	6	0	6
1982	7	3	10
1983	6	3	9
1984	3	0	3
1985	1	1	2
1986	6	1	7
1987	4	3	7
1988	10	0	10
1989	9	2	11
1990	3	3	6
1991	3	1	4
1992	9	1	10
Total	215	56	271

A 21-year-old college player collapsed on the field during preseason drills and died the same day in the hospital. An autopsy report stated that the death was related to sickle cell trait and an enlarged heart.

There were 80 heat stroke deaths in junior/senior high school and college football from 1960 through 1992. As illustrated in Table 3.9 (page 50), 64 were in junior/senior high school football and 16 in college football. In 1970, there

Table 3.6   Indirect Football Fatalities Rate per 100,000, 1960-1992

Year	High school	College	Year	High school	College
1960	0.32	3.04	1977	0.40	0.00
1961	1.79	0.00	1978	0.53	1.33
1962	0.65	3.04	1979	0.53	1.33
1963	0.65	3.04	1980	0.31	0.00
1964	2.00	1.52	1981	0.46	1.33
1965	1.40	6.67	1982	0.54	1.33
1966	0.60	2.67	1983	0.46	4.00
1967	0.40	1.33	1984	0.23	0.00
1968	0.80	2.67	1985	0.08	1.33
1969	0.73	4.00	1986	0.46	1.33
1970	1.00	2.67	1987	0.31	4.00
1971	0.58	2.67	1988	0.77	0.00
1972	0.83	1.33	1989	0.60	2.67
1973	0.42	4.00	1990	0.20	4.00
1974	0.42	4.00	1991	0.20	1.33
1975	0.25	4.00	1992	0.60	1.33
1976	0.47	2.67			

Participation numbers have changed over the years and these changes are reflected in the yearly rates. Since 1989, the participation numbers are 1,500,000 for senior and junior high schools and 75,000 for colleges.

Table 3.7   Indirect Football Fatalities: Type Injury, High School 1960-1992

Injury	Number	Percentage
Heart attack	97	45.1
Heat stroke	64	29.8
Complications	10	4.6
Aneurysm	9	4.2
Sickle cell	4	1.9
Asthma	4	1.9
Other	10	4.6
Unknown	17	7.9
Total	215	100.0

were eight heat stroke deaths in football, the highest number since data collection was started in 1931. There were no heat stroke fatalities from 1931 through 1954 and only five from 1955 through 1959.

Table 3.8   Indirect Football Fatalities: Type Injury, College 1960-1992

Injury	Number	Percentage
Heart attack	18	32.1
Heat stroke	16	28.6
Complications	6	10.7
Sickle cell	5	8.9
Aneurysm	3	5.4
Other	2	3.6
Unknown	6	10.7
Total	56	100.0

Table 3.9   Heat Stroke Fatalities: High School and College Football, 1960-1992

Year	Total	Year	Total
1960	3	1977	1
1961	3	1978	4
1962	5	1979	2
1963	0	1980	1
1964	4	1981	2
1965	6	1982	2
1966	1	1983	1
1967	2	1984	3
1968	5	1985	0
1969	5	1986	0
1970	8	1987	1
1971	4	1988	2
1972	7	1989	1
1973	3	1990	1
1974	1	1991	0
1975	0	1992	1
1976	1	Total	80

High school: 64; college: 16.

Why did heat stroke deaths begin in the late 1950s and cause the death of 80 junior/senior high school and college athletes between 1960 and 1992? Although there are no scientific data to support a reliable answer, it is a fact that water was withheld from football athletes during practice and games in hot weather during the 1960s and 1970s. Coaches felt that giving water to athletes hindered their fitness level and that withholding water made them tough. Of course, this is not true, and this perception was the direct cause of many heat-related fatalities.

In 1970, there were eight heat stroke deaths. The number of heat stroke deaths has been reduced, but there is a continuing problem with heat-related illness and death. From 1987 through 1992, there was an average of one heat stroke death each year. Heat stroke deaths in football are preventable if proper precautions are taken.

Disability Injuries (1977-1992)

Catastrophic or disability injuries are defined as those resulting in brain and spinal cord injury or skull and spine fracture. All cases involve some disability at the time of the injury. Neurological recovery is either complete or incomplete (quadriplegia or quadriparesis). Annual follow-up is not done, thus neurological status (complete or incomplete recovery) refers to the time at which the athlete is entered into the registry. This is usually 2 or 3 months after the injury.

From 1977 through 1992, as shown in Table 3.10, there were 127 high school and 20 college football players with incomplete neurological recovery from cervical cord injuries, for a total of 147 players. These data indicate a reduction in the number of cervical cord injuries with incomplete recovery when compared to data published in the early 1970s.

Table 3.10   Football Cervical Cord Injuries, 1977-1992, Incomplete Recovery

Year	High school	College	Total
1977	10	2	12
1978	13	0	13
1979	8	3	11
1980	11	2	13
1981	6	2	8
1982	7	2	9
1983	11	1	12
1984	5	0	5
1985	6	3	9
1986	3	0	3
1987	9	0	9
1988	10	1	11
1989	12	2	14
1990	11	2	13
1991	1	0	1
1992	4	0	4
Total	127	20	147

While data from 1988, 1989, and 1990 suggest a gradual increase in these types of injuries, the 1991 data show the most dramatic reduction since the beginning of the study in 1977. There was a slight rise in 1992 to four high school injuries.

As mentioned earlier in this chapter, the latest participation figures available show 1,500,000 players at the junior and senior high school level and 75,000 in college football. Table 3.11 illustrates the incidence of cervical spine injuries with incomplete recovery per 100,000 participants. Both high school and college rates were low, and the junior/senior high school rates were less than one per 100,000 participants. For these 16 years, the high school incidence was .59 per 100,000 participants, and the college incidence was 1.66 per 100,000 participants.

Table 3.12 indicates that when comparing cervical cord injuries between offensive and defensive players, there are many more injuries to defensive players. During the 16-year period from 1977 through 1992, 107 of the 147 players with cervical cord injuries were playing defense and only 22 were playing offense. The following case studies help illustrate this fact:

Case Studies

A 15-year-old high school player fractured cervical vertebrae 5 and 6 in a game. He was playing linebacker and hit a receiver from behind with his head in a slightly flexed position (chin to chest). The athlete had surgery with incomplete neurological recovery.

A 19-year-old high school player sustained a Jefferson fracture of the first cervical vertebra in a tackling drill. The injured athlete was the ball carrier in the drill and made contact with the crown of his helmet to the crown of the tackler's helmet. There was no neurological deficit.

Table 3.11   Football Cervical Cord Injuries Incomplete Recovery Rate per 100,000 Participants, 1977-1992

Year	High school	College	Year	High school	College
1977	0.77	2.67	1985	0.46	4.00
1978	1.00	0.00	1986	0.23	0.00
1979	0.62	4.00	1987	0.69	0.00
1980	0.85	2.67	1988	0.77	1.33
1981	0.46	2.67	1989	0.80	2.67
1982	0.54	2.67	1990	0.73	2.67
1983	0.85	1.33	1991	0.07	0.00
1984	0.38	0.00	1992	0.27	0.00

From 1977-1988 based on 1,300,000 senior and junior high school players and 75,000 college players. In 1989 senior and junior high school figure increased to 1,500,000.

**Table 3.12   Football Cervical Cord Injuries Incomplete Recovery:
Offensive vs. Defensive Football, 1977-1992**

Year	Offensive	Defensive	Unknown	Total
1977	0	7	5	12
1978	1	11	1	13
1979	1	5	5	11
1980	3	8	2	13
1981	3	4	1	8
1982	3	6	0	9
1983	2	10	0	12
1984	1	3	1	5
1985	1	8	0	9
1986	0	3	0	3
1987	1	6	2	9
1988	2	9	0	11
1989	0	13	1	14
1990	2	11	0	13
1991	0	1	0	1
1992	2	2	0	4
Total	22	107	18	147

A 20-year-old college football player was injured while tackling in a spring practice goal-line scrimmage. It was a helmet-to-helmet collision, and the player made initial contact with the crown of his helmet. His recovery was incomplete.

Table 3.13 (page 54) shows that the majority of the defensive players were tackling when injured. Fifty players were recorded as tackling, and 43 were recorded as tackling with their heads down or making initial contact with the crown of the helmet. Another eight were tackling on kick-offs, and four were tackling on punts. Of the 147 players injured, 105 or 71.3% were involved in some type of tackle.

Table 3.14 (page 54) reveals that defensive backs are injured at a higher rate than players in other positions. Of the players with cervical cord injuries, 34.7% were defensive backs. Kick-off team players followed with 10.9% of the injuries, and linebackers were a close third with 10.2%. A typical scenario is a defensive back making a tackle in the open field with the head in a position of flexion.

In 1984, the NCCSIR began to collect data concerning cerebral injuries with incomplete recovery. As shown in Table 3.15 (page 55), from 1984 through 1992 there were 31 cerebral injuries at the junior/senior high school level and 4 at the college level. All of these injuries were subdural hematomas with some type of permanent disability.

Table 3.13   Football Cervical Cord Injuries: Type of Activity, 1977-1992

Activity	Number	Percent
Tackling	50	34.0
Tackling head down	43	29.2
Tackling on punt	4	2.7
Tackling on kick-off	8	5.4
Tackled	12	8.2
Tackled on kick-off	2	1.4
Collision	3	2.0
Blocking on kick	3	2.0
Blocking	0	0.0
Contact after interception	2	1.4
Blocked	2	1.4
Hitting Tacklematic	1	0.7
Unknown	17	11.6
Total	147	100.0

Table 3.14   Football Cervical Cord Injuries: Position Played, 1977-1992

Position	Number	Percent
Defensive back	51	34.7
Kick-off team	16	10.9
Defensive line	8	5.4
Linebacker	15	10.2
Kick-off return	6	4.1
Defensive end	5	3.4
Offensive back	7	4.7
Quarterback	4	2.7
Flanker	2	1.4
Wide receiver	1	0.7
Punt coverage	3	2.0
Punt return	1	0.7
Drill	2	1.4
Offensive line	0	0.0
Unknown	26	17.7
Total	147	100.0

Table 3.15   Football Cerebral Injuries, 1984-1992, Incomplete Recovery

Year	High school	College	Total
1984	5	2	7
1985	4	1	5
1986	2	0	2
1987	2	0	2
1988	4	0	4
1989	6	0	6
1990	2	0	2
1991	3	1	4
1992	3	0	3
Total	31	4	35

In addition to the cervical cord and cerebral injuries with incomplete recovery, there are a number of these injuries with complete recovery. These injuries include fractured cervical vertebrae, transient paralysis due to bruising of the spinal cord, subdural hematomas, and, in a small number of cases, fractured skulls. These injuries are very difficult to track on a national level, but a very rough estimate is approximately double the number of injuries with incomplete recovery. In some of these cases, the participant had excellent medical coverage, and this made the difference between complete and incomplete recovery.

Disability injuries to the head and neck have been reduced since the early 1970s, but they have not been eliminated and may never be. The initial reduction was due to the general concern in the total athletic community, but the major reduction, as in the drop in fatalities, was due to the rule change in 1976 that eliminated use of the head as the initial point of contact during blocking and tackling.

Other important changes were improved medical care of the injured athlete at both the game site and in medical facilities and improved coaching techniques in teaching the fundamentals of tackling and blocking. A concerted effort must be made to continue the reduction of cervical spine injuries to football players and to aim for the elimination of both cervical spine and cerebral injuries.

References

1. Danzig A: *The history of American football.* Englewood Cliffs, NJ: Prentice-Hall; 1956.
2. Mueller FO, Schindler RD: *Annual survey of football injury research.* Orlando, FL: The American Football Coaches Association; 1993.
3. National Collegiate Athletic Association: Overland Park, KS; 1992.
4. American Football Coaches Association: 53rd annual proceedings. Durham, NC; 1976.

Chapter 4

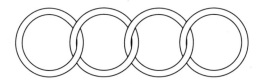

Team Sports

In addition to football, five other team sports have been associated with catastrophic injuries at the high school and college levels—soccer, basketball, ice hockey, baseball, and lacrosse. Each of these sports will be covered in this chapter.

Soccer

Soccer is the most popular sport in the world, and its popularity is gaining in the United States. It has been estimated that there were 22 million soccer players in the world in the early 1980s, and that number is increasing. In the United States soccer is now a major sport at both the high school and college levels.

The National Federation of State High School Associations (NFSHSA) 1993–94 Handbook shows that soccer is the fifth most popular sport for females, with 149,053 participants (1). In only a decade, the number of participants has almost tripled: In 1982-83, girls' soccer was ranked number eight, with 57,921 participants. This is a dramatic increase duplicated in no other sport.

Although the growth has not been as dramatic as in girls' soccer, soccer is also the fifth most popular sport among males, with 242,095 participants. In 1982-83, boys' soccer was ranked seventh, with 162,504 participants.

Soccer's popularity has also been evident at the college level. According to the February 16, 1994, edition of the *NCAA News*, women's soccer showed the largest participation gains in the 1992–93 school year, a 37% increase over the 1991–92 participation numbers (2). There are now 8,226 women playing soccer in National Collegiate Athletic Association (NCAA) colleges and universities. Male soccer at the college level experienced a participation increase of 10% in the 1992–93 school year, which makes soccer the fifth fastest growing sport for men in NCAA colleges and universities. NCAA records show 14,795 male soccer participants in 1992–93.

Due to these dramatic increases in soccer participation in the United States, there is also a concern about soccer injuries. There have not been any national injury studies for soccer at the high school level, but the NCAA has a national injury data collection system for college soccer. Women's NCAA soccer shows a practice injury rate of 5.6 injuries per 1,000 athlete exposures, and a game injury rate of 16.5 injuries per 1,000 athlete exposures from 1987 to 1994. For that same period of time, men's soccer had a practice injury rate of 4.8 injuries per 1,000 athlete exposures and a game injury rate of 20.1 per 1,000 athlete exposures.

Direct Soccer Fatalities (1982-1992)

As illustrated in Table 4.1, high school soccer was associated with two fatalities during the period from 1982 to 1992. One fatality occurred during the 1983–84 school year and the other during the 1990–91 school year. Both fatalities involved male participants.

One case involved a junior varsity goalie who challenged an opposing player's attempt to kick a goal. The opponent's knee struck the goalie in the chest and fractured two ribs. One of the fractured ribs punctured a lung and lacerated the heart. The athlete died from his injuries and was listed as a direct fatality.

The second fatality involved a 15-year-old male high school soccer player who died from head injuries suffered in a game. The player collided with a teammate and struck his head on the field. Cause of death was cerebral trauma.

Soccer participation at the high school level averaged approximately 202,000 males and 94,000 females each year. Table 4.2 shows that the fatality injury rate per 100,000 participants was 0.10 for males and 0.00 for females. The fatality injury rate for males and females combined is 0.07 per 100,000 participants.

Table 4.1   Direct Soccer Fatalities, 1982-1983 to 1991-1992

Year	High school	College	Total
1982-1983	0	0	0
1983-1984	1	0	1
1984-1985	0	0	0
1985-1986	0	0	0
1986-1987	0	0	0
1987-1988	0	0	0
1988-1989	0	0	0
1989-1990	0	0	0
1990-1991	1	0	1
1991-1992	0	0	0
Total	2	0	2

Table 4.2   High School Soccer Direct Fatalities per 100,000 Participants

Athletes	Fatality rate
Male	0.10
Female	0.00
Combined ·	0.07

Table 4.3   Indirect Soccer Fatalities, 1982-1983 to 1991-1992

Year	High school	College	Total
1982-1983	0	0	0
1983-1984	0	0	0
1984-1985	0	0	0
1985-1986	1	0	1
1986-1987	3	0	3
1987-1988	0	0	0
1988-1989	0	0	0
1989-1990	1	0	1
1990-1991	2	0	2
1991-1992	1	0 .	1
Total	8	0	8

The data also show that there were no fatal injuries to males or females at the college level from 1982 to 1992. College annual participation numbers averaged approximately 14,000 men and 5,000 women.

Indirect Soccer Fatalities (1982-1992)

Indirect soccer fatalities numbered eight at the high school level and none at the college level (Table 4.3). All eight fatalities involved male soccer players, and up to 1992 there have been no indirect fatalities to female soccer players. Examples of three indirect fatalities are as follows:

Case Studies

A 17-year-old high school player collapsed after a game while walking off the field. He died later that day at the hospital. The athlete had an asthma attack and died from cardiac arrest.

A 17-year-old high school player collapsed during a game and died from cardiac arrest. He had a heart murmur but had had medical clearance to play.

A 13-year-old high school player collapsed and died during practice. The athlete had a known congenital heart problem, but he and his family decided that he would play nevertheless. Cause of death was listed as idiopathic left ventricular hypertrophy.

The indirect fatality rate for males at the high school level was 0.40 per 100,000 participants. If males and females are combined, the rate is 0.27 per 100,000 participants (Table 4.4).

A major concern in soccer has been catastrophic injuries to participants and children caused by the movable soccer goals falling over and causing death or disability. A release by the Consumer Product Safety Commission on September 30, 1992, provided information about 15 deaths and several serious injuries since 1979 resulting from soccer goal tip-overs. The victims ranged in age from 3 to 22 years. The typical accident happened when someone climbed on or hung from a soccer goal that was not anchored. The goal fell over and crushed this individual.

Soccer Serious Injuries (1982-1992)

As shown in Table 4.5, there were only four serious injuries in high school soccer in these 10 years, and all four participants recovered or were expected to recover completely. All four injuries were to male participants. One case involved a freshman player who was knocked unconscious during a play-off game. He crashed into a chain linked fence surrounding the field while battling for the ball, and suffered a fractured tailbone and a bruised head. A full recovery was expected.

The injury rate for serious injuries was 0.20 for male participants; thus, for the combined male and female number the serious injury rate would be 0.13 per 100,000 participants (Table 4.6). There was only one catastrophic injury at the college level, and that was also a serious injury with full recovery.

An interesting study of serious soccer injuries was conducted by the Department of Neurosurgery and Psychosomatic Medicine at the National Hospital in Oslo, Norway, and published in 1991 (3). Thirty-seven former soccer players of the National Football Team in Norway were examined with a battery of psychological tests. Eighty-one percent of the players demonstrated mild to severe deficits regarding attention, concentration, memory, and judgment. The researcher concluded that this may indicate some degree of permanent organic brain damage from the cumulative result of repeated traumas from heading the ball.

Table 4.4   High School Soccer Indirect Fatalities per 100,000 Participants

Athletes	Fatality rate
Male	0.40
Female	0.00
Combined	0.27

Table 4.5   Soccer Serious Injuries,* 1982-1983 to 1991-1992

Year	High school	College	Total
1982-1983	1	0	1
1983-1984	0	0	0
1984-1985	1	0	1
1985-1986	0	0	0
1986-1987	0	1	1
1987-1988	0	0	0
1988-1989	0	0	0
1989-1990	0	0	0
1990-1991	1	0	1
1991-1992	1	0	1
Total	4	1	5

*Serious injuries are defined as possible disability injuries but with complete recovery.

Table 4.6   High School and College Soccer Serious Injuries per 100,000 Participants

Athletes	High school	College
Male	0.20	0.70
Female	0.00	0.00
Combined	0.13	0.51

Basketball

Basketball was invented in the United States in 1891, and its popularity has grown ever since. It is played around the world, and can be seen from the playgrounds of the United States to the Olympic Games. The NFSHSA ranks basketball as the most popular sport for both males and females, with 16,462 schools sponsoring boys' basketball and 15,864 schools sponsoring girls' basketball. Boys' basketball ranks second to football with 515,423 participants, and girls' basketball ranks first, with 387,802 participants. For the 10-year period from 1982–83 through 1991–92, 5,113,733 males and 3,907,964 females participated in high school basketball. College basketball is also very popular, and for that same period of time there were 128,018 male and 106,129 female basketball participants. There are 827 NCAA colleges and universities that sponsor women's basketball—more college participation than any other women's sport. Indeed, women's basketball has grown at a phenomenal rate since Title IX legislation was enacted in 1972.

With this great increase in participation, injuries are always a concern. As in most sports at the high school level, non-catastrophic injury data are not available. The NCAA's national injury database shows that women's basketball ranks 9th in practice injuries and 11th in game injuries when compared with 16 other sports (4).

The practice injury rate was 4.09 per 1,000 athlete exposures as compared to football spring practice at 9.18 and women's gymnastics at 7.22. The game injury rate for women's basketball was 8.95 per 1,000 athlete exposures as compared to football at 36.20 and women's gymnastics at 21.26. The ankle and the knee are the body parts injured most often, and most injuries are not considered serious.

Direct Basketball Fatalities (1982-1992)

Direct fatality data collected for all sports at both the high school and college levels indicate that both high school and college basketball are risk free for males and females. For the 10-year period from 1982 to 1992, there were no direct fatalities in high school or college basketball.

Indirect Basketball Fatalities (1982-1992)

As shown in Table 4.7, there have been a number of indirect basketball fatalities at both the high school and college levels. For the 10-year period we have been discussing, there were 37 indirect deaths at the high school level, and all 37 were heart related. Thirty-five of the fatalities were to males and two involved females. Sixteen of the fatalities happened in games and 21 at practice. The 10-year indirect fatality rate for high school males was 0.68 per 100,000 participants and

Table 4.7   Indirect Basketball Fatalities, 1982-1983 to 1991-1992

Year	High school	College	Total
1982-1983	4	1	5
1983-1984	3	1	4
1984-1985	3	0	3
1985-1986	1	0	1
1986-1987	3	0	3
1987-1988	4	3	7
1988-1989	2	1	3
1989-1990	4	1	5
1990-1991	7	0	7
1991-1992	6	1	7
Total	37	8	45

Table 4.8   Basketball Indirect Fatalities per 100,000 Participants

Athletes	Fatality rate	
	High school	College
Male	0.68	5.47
Female	0.05	0.94
Combined	0.41	3.42

0.05 for high school females (Table 4.8). This fatality rate is not high, but when 37 high school athletes have heart-related deaths, there is cause for concern.

College basketball was also associated with eight indirect fatalities—seven males and one female. All eight were heart-related, with two happening in games, four in practice, and two unknown. The 10-year fatality rate for college males was 5.47 per 100,000 participants, and 0.94 for college females. The rate for college males is high and should be of concern.

As is true in all sports, indirect fatalities in basketball involve collapse: An athlete collapses either on the court in a game or practice, on the sideline, or in the locker room. Following are case reports of indirect fatalities:

Case Studies

A 17-year-old high school player collapsed and died after a 2-hr practice. Cause of death was hypertrophic cardiomyopathy. The athlete had no history of cardiac problems.

A 16-year-old high school player collapsed and died while running three man weave drills in practice. Mitral valve prolapse had been diagnosed by a cardiologist and physician during the medical examination.

A 15-year-old high school basketball player collapsed and died during practice. Cause of death was related to a defective coronary artery.

Basketball Disability and Serious Injuries (1982-1992)

As shown in Table 4.9 (page 64), high school basketball was associated with four catastrophic injuries from 1982 to 1992. Two of the injuries involved permanent disability, and two of the injuries were serious. One of the disability injuries involved a female player being hit with an elbow in the throat, which injured the larynx; the second one took place when a male player collided with a teammate and hit a wall, fracturing a cervical vertebra.

The two serious injuries involved a spinal contusion and a fractured cervical vertebra. In high school basketball, the injury rates per 100,000 participants were very low, as shown in Table 4.10 (page 64).

Table 4.9   Basketball Catastrophic Injuries, 1982-1983 to 1991-1992

Year	High school	College	Total
1982-1983	0	0	0
1983-1984	0	0	0
1984-1985	1	0	1
1985-1986	0	1	1
1986-1987	0	0	0
1987-1988	1	0	1
1988-1989	2	1	3
1989-1990	0	0	0
1990-1991	0	0	0
1991-1992	0	0	0
Total	4	2	6

Table 4.10   High School and College Basketball Catastrophic Injuries per 100,000 Participants

Athletes	High school	College
Male	0.06	1.56
Female	0.03	0.00
Combined	0.04	0.85

College basketball during this same 10-year period was associated with two serious injuries. One injury was a fractured cervical vertebra and the second was a severe concussion. Both injuries happened during collisions. As shown in Tables 4.9 and 4.10, direct catastrophic injuries in college basketball were also low in number.

Ice Hockey

Ice hockey is a popular sport in the United States, but its popularity is limited to certain geographical locations. Canada is recognized as the birthplace of ice hockey, where it is considered the national sport. According to 1985 participation figures, there are over 500,000 amateur players in Canada (5).

Participation figures are not that high in the United States, where annual high school participation averaged approximately 23,000 and college participation averaged 4,000 during the period from 1982-83 to 1991-92.

A closer look at the high school participation figures shows that ice hockey was not listed in the 10 most popular sports by either males or females. In fact, the number of male participants declined, although there was an increase in female ice hockey players. In the 1982–83 school year, there were 23,970 males and 49 females, while in 1991–92 there were 22,116 males and 120 females. Most of the females participated as members of the male teams.

It is interesting to note that despite this decrease in participants, there was a slight increase in the number of schools playing ice hockey. School participation increased from 823 in 1982–83 to 925 in 1991–92.

The rise in female participation may continue as schools continue to comply with Title IX legislation. In March of 1994, the Minnesota State High School League's Representative Assembly voted to sanction girls' high school ice hockey beginning with the 1994–95 season (6). Another reason for the continued interest in ice hockey by females is the fact that women's ice hockey will be a full medal sport at the 1998 Winter Olympics.

College ice hockey suffered a similar overall decrease in participation figures for the 10-year period mentioned above. In 1982–83, there were 3,927 male participants on 123 teams and 359 female participants on 17 teams. The numbers for 1991–92 show a decrease to 3,663 males on 121 teams.

Information for females was not available because this information is not recorded if there are fewer than 10 teams participating. However, with the expected increase in high school female participation and with further participation increased due to Title IX and the 1998 Olympics, college figures will probably rise during the next decade.

Because ice hockey is a fast-paced contact sport that can at times be considered violent, there is concern for the safety of the participants. Between 1966 and 1987, there were 112 reported cases of major spinal cord injury in Canada, and between 1982 and 1986 up to 15 cases of major spinal cord injury to Canadian ice hockey players (7). Most of these injuries were to teenagers and to players under 30 years of age playing in supervised games.

Although there are no data to support this at the present time, a number of researchers think that the high number of spinal cord injuries in ice hockey is related to the addition of the face mask. They believe that the face mask has altered the nature of the game, giving players a feeling of invincibility that leads to taking unwarranted risks. According to a recent article in the *NCAA News*, the 1981 mandate for use of the full face mask in college ice hockey has changed the game from one played below the waist to one played above the waist, with the result that it has become faster and more physical (8).

Again, the injury data do not support these statements. However, injury data do support the fact that the use of the helmet and full face mask has decreased the number of facial and eye injuries. The lack of adequate ice hockey injury data has been a major problem.

Direct Ice Hockey Fatalities (1982-1992)

As shown in Table 4.11 (page 66), there was only one direct fatality in both high school and college ice hockey during this time. This fatality happened in high school hockey to a 15-year-old 10th-grader in a varsity game.

Table 4.11   Direct Ice Hockey Fatalities, 1982-1983 to 1991-1992

Year	High school	College	Total
1982-1983	0	0	0
1983-1984	0	0	0
1984-1985	0	0	0
1985-1986	0	0	0
1986-1987	0	0	0
1987-1988	0	0	0
1988-1989	1	0	1
1989-1990	0	0	0
1990-1991	0	0	0
1991-1992	0	0	0
Total	1	0	1

The injured player had the puck in the opponents' zone, and was knocked to the ice by an opponent. As he fell to the ice, a teammate shot the puck, which struck him in the left chest area. Due to the position of the injured player, a small portion of his chest was not covered by the protective equipment. The blow to the chest caused cardiac damage and led to immediate death.

This is the only direct fatality recorded for high school and college hockey for the 10-year period mentioned, but a 16-year-old non-school player was killed in 1991 when he was struck in the head and neck by a puck. He was a goalie and was wearing a face mask, protective collar, and chest guard.

The fatality injury rate for high school males for the period from 1982–83 to 1991–92 was 0.43 per 100,000 participants. Due to the small number of female participants, that rate remains the same if the number of males and females is combined (Table 4.12). As previously indicated, there were no fatal direct injuries in college hockey.

Indirect Ice Hockey Fatalities and Indirect Catastrophic Injuries (1982-1992)

Table 4.13 shows that there were a total of three indirect high school and college ice hockey catastrophic injuries from 1992–83 to 1991–92. One was at the high school level and two were at the college level.

Table 4.12   High School Ice Hockey Direct Fatalities per 100,000 Participants

Athletes	Fatality rate
Male	0.43
Female	0.00
Combined	0.43

Table 4.13   Indirect Ice Hockey Fatalities and Catastrophic Injuries, 1982-1983 to 1991-1992

Year	High school	College	Total
1982-1983	0	0	0
1983-1984	0	1	1
1984-1985	0	0	0
1985-1986	0	0	0
1986-1987	0	0	0
1987-1988	0	0	0
1988-1989	0	0	0
1989-1990	0	0	0
1990-1991	1	0	1
1991-1992	0	1*	1*
Total	1	2	3

*Not a fatality but an indirect catastrophic injury.

Table 4.14   High School and College Ice Hockey Indirect Fatalities per 100,000 Participants

Athletes	High school	College*
Male	0.43	2.48
Female	0.00	0.00
Combined	0.43	2.41

*Rate for college indirect nonfatal = 2.48.

In the high school fatality, the athlete collapsed on the ice during a match and was pronounced dead later that day at the hospital. Cause of death was heart related.

In the one college fatality, the player suffered cardiac arrest during practice and died at the hospital. The college indirect catastrophic injury involved a preseason training exercise where the players participated in a 10K road race during the month of September. The injured athlete collapsed from dehydration during the race and suffered heat stroke. He was hospitalized and had to have both liver and kidney transplants.

The indirect fatal injury rates were 0.43 per 100,000 participants at the high school level and 2.48 at the college level (Table 4.14).

Ice Hockey Disability Injuries (1982-1992)

In this 10-year period, there were four catastrophic disability injuries at the high school level (Table 4.15, page 68). All four injuries happened in games, and all

Table 4.15   Ice Hockey Catastrophic Injuries, 1982-1983 to 1991-1992

Year	High school	College	Total
1982-1983	0	0	0
1983-1984	1	0	1
1984-1985	0	0	0
1985-1986	0	0	0
1986-1987	2	0	2
1987-1988	0	0	0
1988-1989	0	1	1
1989-1990	0	0	0
1990-1991	1	0	1
1991-1992	0	0	0
Total	4	1	5

involved males. As is true in most ice hockey injuries, all four athletes hit the boards head first, fractured one or more cervical vertebrae, and suffered paralysis.

The one college disability injury had circumstances identical to the high school injuries, with the only difference being that the injury took place in a practice session. As the following cases show, almost all ice hockey catastrophic injuries have the same etiology:

Case Studies

A 19-year-old college player fractured his fifth cervical vertebra in a practice scoring drill. He tried to avoid the goalie, fell and slid on his stomach, and hit the boards with the top of his head. He was wearing a helmet and a face mask. The player is now quadriplegic.

An 18-year-old male high school player fractured his neck when he fell head first into the boards during a game. There was no body contact. The player is now quadriplegic.

A 15-year-old male high school player slid head first into the boards after being hit by an opposing player. He fractured cervical vertebrae and is now quadriplegic.

Table 4.16 shows that the high school disability injury rate per 100,000 participants was 1.73. This rate is not only higher than the high school football rate; it is higher than the rates of all of the other winter and spring sports. The college disability injury rate was 2.48 per 100,000 participants.

Ice Hockey Serious Injuries (1982-1992)

In addition to the catastrophic disability injuries, there were six serious ice hockey injuries. Three were at the high school level and three were at the college level

Table 4.16   High School and College Ice Hockey Catastrophic Injuries per 100,000 Participants

Athletes	High school	College
Male	1.73	2.48
Female	0.00	0.00
Combined	1.72	2.41

Table 4.17   Serious Ice Hockey Injuries, 1982-1983 to 1991-1992

Year	High school	College	Total
1982-1983	1	0	1
1983-1984	0	0	0
1984-1985	0	0	0
1985-1986	0	0	0
1986-1987	0	1	1
1987-1988	1	0	1
1988-1989	0	0	0
1989-1990	0	0	0
1990-1991	0	1	1
1991-1992	1	1	2
Total	3	3	6

Table 4.18   High School and College Ice Hockey Serious Injuries per 100,000 Participants

Athletes	High school	College
Male	1.30	7.45
Female	0.00	0.00
Combined	1.29	7.21

(Table 4.17). Two of the high school injuries involved hitting the boards head first, and the third happened when the athlete was struck in the head by the puck in a game. Two accidents took place in games and one in a practice.

One of the college serious injuries involved a 19-year-old college player who fractured three cervical vertebrae during a practice session. He was involved in a four on four drill, and was hit from the side by an opponent. He hit head first into the boards. The athlete had complete recovery. The second injured player also received a neck injury, and the third player had a subdural hematoma with recovery.

The high school serious injury rate was 1.30 injuries per 100,000 participants, but the college injury rate climbs to 7.45 injuries per 100,000 participants (Table 4.18, page 69).

Baseball

Baseball has been very popular in the United States, and every summer about 5 million amateur young men and women participate in organized play. This does not include softball and recreational play. Although baseball has always been rightfully considered a safe game, attention has recently focused on the game's association with fatalities to the participants.

This was highlighted in the television show "60 Minutes," which created public concern. The show emphasized data from the Consumer Product Safety Commission stating that there were 51 baseball-related deaths from 1973 to 1983 that involved ball impact to the chest. Of those 51 deaths, 17 occurred in organized games or practices, 11 in informal play, and 23 in undetermined types of play. The Consumer Product Safety Commission also estimated 86,500 hospital emergency room-treated injuries to children from 5 to 14 years of age in organized baseball.

This concern has continued, and USA Baseball, the governing body of amateur baseball in the United States, has started to collect amateur baseball injury data on a national level. They began with catastrophic data and are expanding the data collection system to include all injuries. A national sample is being used, and the data can be extrapolated to give a reliable picture of the injury problem in amateur baseball in the United States.

High school baseball participation has increased over the 10-year period from 1982–83 to 1992–93. In 1982–83, there were 409,970 male participants and 590 female participants in 13,380 schools across the country. Baseball was ranked as the fourth most popular sport for males.

In 1991–92, the number of males increased to 433,684. The number of participating schools also increased to 13,722, and baseball continued to be ranked as the fourth most popular male sport at the high school level.

Due to their increased participation in softball, the numbers of females decreased to 541 in 1991–92. Softball is not included in the data because there were no catastrophic injuries. With the increased participation, however, there is no doubt that future data collection will include softball—both fast and slow pitch. Fast pitch softball ranks as the fourth most popular high school female sport.

College baseball participation figures show 19,220 athletes in 650 schools during the 1983 baseball season. There was a slight increase in the ensuing 10 years, and during the 1992 season the participation number increased to 21,204 in 713 schools. Softball also showed a dramatic increase at the college level during this period, but there were no catastrophic injuries.

Direct Baseball Fatalities (1982-1992)

As illustrated in Table 4.19, there were three direct fatalities at the high school level during the 10-year period indicated. Two fatalities occurred during the 1984 season to male participants in a practice session and the third in a 1991 practice session. All three injuries involved being hit in the head with a ball, one with a fly ball, the second with a ball thrown by a pitching machine, and the third with a ball hit during outfield practice.

All injuries were diagnosed as subdural hematomas. The athlete hit by the fly ball died 5 days after the accident, the two other athletes died that same day. As shown in Table 4.20, the catastrophic injury rate for high school direct fatalities was 0.07 per 100,000 participants.

There were also two direct deaths at the college level during this period. One death occurred in the spring of 1986 and the second in the spring of 1991. Both injuries occurred in practice situations.

Table 4.19   High School Baseball Direct Catastrophic Injuries, 1982-1983 to 1991-1992

Year	Fatalities	Disability	Serious
1982-1983	0	1	2
1983-1984	2	0	0
1984-1985	0	0	0
1985-1986	0	1	3
1986-1987	0	0	0
1987-1988	0	1	0
1988-1989	0	2	1
1989-1990	0	2	0
1990-1991	1	0	0
1991-1992	0	0	0
Total	3	7	6

Table 4.20   High School Baseball Direct Catastrophic Injuries per 100,000 Participants, 1982-1983 to 1991-1992

Athletes	Fatalities	Disability	Serious
Male	0.07	0.17	0.15
Female	0.00	0.00	0.00
Combined	0.07	0.17	0.15

One of the athletes was hit in the chest with a thrown ball, which caused cardiac arrest. The athlete died the same day. The second athlete collided with another outfielder while chasing a fly ball and died from a head injury 3 days later.

The college injury rate for direct fatalities was 0.89 per 100,000 participants. Additional information concerning fatalities is as follows:

Case Studies

An 18-year-old college player died during pregame drills. He was fielding and throwing ground balls when he was struck in the chest with another thrown ball. He collapsed on the field and died later at the hospital.

A 15-year-old high school player died after being hit in the head with a batted ball while assisting a coach who was hitting balls to the outfielders. The athlete, who was not wearing a helmet, was hit on the side of the head. Cause of death was severe brain damage.

Indirect Baseball Fatalities (1982-1992)

Table 4.21 shows five indirect baseball fatalities at the high school level from the spring of 1983 through the spring of 1992. Four of the fatalities were heart related, with three occurring in games and one in practice. The fifth indirect fatality occurred when the athlete was leaving the field after practice and was struck by lightning.

Two of the athletes with the heart-related deaths collapsed during games, one collapsed while sitting in the dugout, and one while running laps in practice. The indirect fatality injury rate, as shown in Table 4.22, was 0.12 per

Table 4.21   High School and College Indirect Baseball Fatalities, 1982-1983 to 1991-1992

Year	High school	College
1982-1983	0	0
1983-1984	0	0
1984-1985	2	0
1985-1986	0	0
1986-1987	0	0
1987-1988	0	1
1988-1989	1	0
1989-1990	1	0
1990-1991	1	0
1991-1992	0	1
Total	5	2

Table 4.22   High School and College Indirect Baseball Fatality Rate per 100,000 Participants, 1982-1983 to 1991-1992

Athletes	High school	College
Male	0.12	0.98
Female	0.00	0.00
Combined	0.12	0.98

100,000 participants. Injury rates for both direct and indirect fatalities are low for high school baseball.

College baseball was associated with two indirect fatalities from 1983 to 1992. Both fatalities were heart related, with one taking place during conditioning drills and the second in the training room. Both athletes collapsed during the activity they were involved in, and both died the same day.

Table 4.22 shows the indirect fatality rate for college baseball to be 0.98 per 100,000 participants. The college rate was slightly higher than the high school rate, but both were less than one per 100,000.

Baseball Disability Injuries (1982-1992)

As illustrated in Table 4.19 (page 71), there were seven permanent disability injuries to high school baseball players from the spring of 1983 through the spring of 1992. Four of the injuries involved the head and three involved the neck. Five of the injuries occurred in games and two in practice.

Catastrophic baseball injuries usually happen in one of three ways—a player is hit by the ball, collides with another player, or is hurt in a head first slide. In looking at the seven disability injuries, this holds true. Three of the injuries happened with the head first slide. Two of the players were sliding into home plate and one into third base. Injuries with the head first slide occur when the base runner hits the top of his head into the leg of the opponent or into the base, causing axial loading on the cervical spine and either a fracture or dislocation of the cervical vertebrae.

Three of the injuries occurred with two players on the same team chasing a fly ball and colliding with a teammate. The last disability injury occurred when the injured athlete was struck in the head with a line drive during batting practice. The injured player was the pitcher and batting practice was taking place in a batting cage. The injured player had a protective screen but was not wearing a batting helmet. Two case studies follow:

Case Studies

A 16-year-old high school baseball player was advancing to third base on a batted ball and slid head first. His head collided with the third baseman and he fractured his fifth cervical vertebra. The athlete is now quadriplegic.

A 16-year-old high school baseball player received a catastrophic head injury in a practice session. The injured player was running back for a fly ball from his second base position. He collided with the right fielder who was running in to catch the fly ball. The player received a head injury with brain damage and permanent disability.

For the 10-year period indicated in Table 4.20 (page 71), the injury rate per 100,000 participants for disability injuries to high school baseball players was 0.17.

During this same period of time college baseball was not associated with any permanent disability injuries.

Baseball Serious Injuries (1982-1992)

In addition to the fatalities and disability injuries, high school baseball was associated with six serious injuries (Table 4.19, page 71). Serious injuries involve the same types of activity and injury but do not include permanent disability. The high school serious injuries included four injuries to the head and two to the neck.

Four of the injuries occurred in games and two in practice. Three of them involved the collision of two players chasing a fly ball, two occurred with the head first slide into home plate, and one took place when the player was struck in the head by a batted ball during batting practice. The player was standing behind the mound and was not wearing a batting helmet. As shown in Table 4.20 (page 71), the serious injury rate for high school baseball players was 0.15 per 100,000 participants.

College baseball was associated with one serious injury during this same time span. The injured player was hit in the head by a batted ball in practice and suffered a fractured skull with full recovery. The player was the batting practice pitcher and was pitching from behind a batting screen. The serious injury rate for college baseball players per 100,000 participants was 0.49.

Lacrosse

Lacrosse was invented by Native Americans, making it the oldest American sport. Native Americans enjoyed the game for the competition, but also used it as a training school for war. The skill, strength, stamina, and speed required to play provided excellent training for the warriors. For a long time, lacrosse was played primarily at a small number of northeastern colleges and prep schools, but recently it has enjoyed a rapid expansion, and many other schools and colleges have initiated play.

High school participation figures from the 1982–83 school year show 15,777 males playing in 272 schools and 6,365 females playing in 161 schools across the country. These numbers are not large compared to the approximately 1,000,000 football players every year. In the 1991–92 school year, the male participation level increased to 20,883 in 413 schools, and female participation to 10,544 in 258 schools. These numbers still cannot compare to some of the more popular sports, but the increase has been substantial.

College participation figures in 1982–83 show 4,519 males in 138 schools and 2,887 females in 113 schools. In 1991–92, these numbers increased to 5,086 males in 160 schools and 2,858 females in 122 schools. The increase was not very dramatic; indeed, female participation actually dropped by 29 athletes even as the number of schools increased by nine. Because many schools and colleges across the country are providing more opportunities for females due to Title IX, lacrosse may well become the sport of choice.

One would think that lacrosse would be associated with a large number of catastrophic injuries because it is a body contact sport. In addition, at the high school level, a number of football players have started to play the game because it is played in the spring and is a good out-of-season activity. With the participation of football players, lacrosse could have become a more violent sport.

However, the rule makers were ahead of the game, disallowing use of the head in initial contact and introducing a more protective helmet. Moreover, coaches realized that the better teams were skilled in ball and stick handling. Whether these changes are responsible for this or not, lacrosse has not been associated with a high number of catastrophic injuries.

Direct Lacrosse Fatalities (1982-1992)

As mentioned in the introduction, lacrosse catastrophic injuries are fairly rare. From 1982 to 1992, there was only one direct fatality in high school and college lacrosse. This fatality was associated with high school lacrosse and happened in the spring of 1987.

It is interesting to note that the injury happened the same way a football injury would have taken place. The 17-year-old high school player ran into an opposing player with his head down and made contact with the top or crown of the helmet. He fractured a cervical vertebra, was paralyzed from the chest down, and died from injury complications 1 month after the accident.

The high school direct fatality rate per 100,000 participants was 0.57 for males and 0.39 for males and females combined. There were no college direct deaths.

Indirect Lacrosse Fatalities (1982-1992)

From the spring of 1982 through the spring of 1992 there were two indirect fatalities in lacrosse, one at the high school level and one at the college level. The high school indirect fatality took place in a game when an inactive player collapsed on the field. Cause of death was heart related. The high school indirect fatality rate per 100,000 participants was 0.57 for males and 0.39 for males and females combined.

The college indirect fatality was also heart related, and took place during out-of-season practice in the fall semester. No other information was available due to litigation. The college indirect fatality rate per 100,000 participants was 2.05 for males and 1.27 for males and females combined.

Disability and Serious Injuries (1982-1992)

High school lacrosse was not associated with any catastrophic disability or serious injuries during this period, while college lacrosse was associated with three catastrophic lacrosse injuries. Two of the injuries were disability injuries, and one was considered serious. The serious injury involved a 20-year-old player who fractured a cervical vertebra during a face-off in a game. The athlete charged into a face-off scramble with his head down, striking another player with the top or crown of his helmet. The player made a full recovery from his injuries.

One of the disability injuries, involving a fractured cervical vertebra, occurred when the athlete was thrown to the ground by an opponent and landed on his neck during a game. The second disability injury involved a female athlete being hit in the eye by a shot. Her eye socket was shattered and she received permanent vision problems.

Women's lacrosse is experiencing a period of controversy regarding the lacrosse helmet. At present, the women's game does not require that players wear a helmet. However, there is a group that is in favor of making the wearing of the helmet mandatory. Those opposed believe that if players wear helmets, the game will change and involve more body contact, becoming more like the men's game. If the helmet is mandated, only time will tell how the game will change.

The college disability injury rate per 100,000 participants was 2.05 for males, 3.35 for females, and 2.54 for males and females combined. The serious injury rate per 100,000 participants was 2.05 for males and 1.27 for males and females combined.

References

1. National Federation of State High School Associations: *1993-1994 Handbook*. Kansas City, MO; 1993.
2. National Collegiate Athletic Association: *NCAA News*. Overland Park, KS; February 16, 1994.
3. Tysvaer AT, Lochen EA: Soccer injuries to the brain. *Am J Sports Med.* Jan.-Feb. 1991;19:(no 1).
4. National Collegiate Athletic Association: *NCAA athletic injury surveillance system*. Overland Park, KS; 1993.
5. Schneider RC, Bull C, et al: *Sports injuries: mechanisms, prevention and treatment*. Baltimore: Williams and Wilkins; 1985.
6. Cohen A: Icewomen cometh. *Athletic Business*. November 1993
7. Tator CH, et al: National survey of spinal injuries in hockey players. *Can Med Assoc J*. April 1984; 130.
8. Breidenthal TA: Geared up: hockey examines equipment's safety value. *NCAA News*. February 9, 1994.

Chapter 5

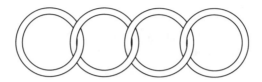

Individual Sports

Five individual competition sports were associated with catastrophic injuries at the high school and college levels—gymnastics, swimming, wrestling, track and field, and cheerleading. Each of these sports will be covered in this chapter.

Gymnastics

Gymnastics is one of the few sports that has shown a reduction in the number of participants during the past decade. During the 1982–83 school year, gymnastics was ranked number nine among girls, and was not among the 10 most popular sports for boys. In that same year, there were 45,736 female and 9,325 male high school participants.

Ten years later, in the 1992–93 school year, gymnastics was not ranked in the top 10 most popular sports for either boys or girls. In 1992–93, the number of female participants numbered 21,216, a dramatic reduction of 24,520 participants when compared to the 1982–83 data. In that same year, the number of male participants decreased to 2,939, a drop of 6,386 participants.

One explanation for this reduction in high school participation figures is that the number of participants at the club level has risen dramatically along with the number of younger participants (1). Gymnastics can also be a very expensive sport when all of the equipment is taken into consideration. It is also quite obvious that with all of the difficult skills involved in gymnastics, it would not be easy for a high school to hire a qualified coach.

College gymnastics also had dramatic reductions in participation levels from 1982–83 to 1992–93. Male college participants numbered 1,569 in 1982–83, and that number dropped to 590 in 1992–93, with only 40 schools sponsoring the sport. Women's gymnastics did not do any better, with the number of participants decreasing from 1,934 in 1982–83 to 1,200 in 1992–93. The reduction of participants at the college level has been so dramatic that the National Collegiate

Athletic Association (NCAA) is considering not having a national championship in men's gymnastics.

With the increased number of gymnastics participants at the club level and with the higher level of difficulty of the skills involved, it is apparent that injury research on club gymnastics is needed.

Direct Gymnastics Fatalities (1982-1992)

Fatalities in high school and college gymnastics are rare, as is shown in Table 5.1. The only fatal injury at the high school level occurred during the 1987–88 school year. A 17-year-old high school gymnast died from injuries received in a fall from the parallel bars during practice.

Male participation at the high school level averaged 5,700 per year, and the fatality injury rate for male high school gymnasts during this 10-year period was 1.75 per 100,000 participants. Female participation averaged approximately 30,000 per year during this time. The combined fatality injury rate for males and females combined is 0.27 per 100,000 participants (Table 5.2).

Table 5.1   Direct Gymnastics Fatalities, 1982-1983 to 1991-1992

Year	High school	College	Total
1982-1983	0	0	0
1983-1984	0	0	0
1984-1985	0	0	0
1985-1986	0	0	0
1986-1987	0	0	0
1987-1988	1	0	1
1988-1989	0	0	0
1989-1990	0	0	0
1990-1991	0	0	0
1991-1992	0	0	0
Total	1	0	1

Table 5.2   High School Gymnastics Direct Fatalities per 100,000 Participants

Athletes	Fatality rate
Male	1.75
Female	0.00
Combined	0.27

There were no college fatalities from 1982 to 1992. In these years, college participation numbers averaged approximately 800 males and 1,600 females each year. As indicated in the introduction, these participation figures are decreasing each year.

Indirect Gymnastics Fatalities (1982-1992)

Gymnastics was the only high school and college sport that did not have any indirect deaths at either level.

Gymnastics Disability Injuries (1982-1992)

Disability injuries at the high school level numbered five for the period indicated above (Table 5.3). Four of the injuries were to female participants and one to a male. All five of the injuries involved permanent disability.

The male gymnast fell off the high bar during a meet and fractured a thoracic vertebra. Two of the female participants were injured while performing on the uneven bars—one in practice and one in a meet. In one injury, a ninth-grade student crushed her 12th thoracic vertebra when attempting a back straddle jump over the high bar from a stand on the low bar of the parallel bars. She fell to the mat on her head and neck and has permanent disability.

In another, a 17-year-old high school gymnast fell from the uneven bars and landed on her neck and back. She was practicing a straddle sole circle 1/2 turn from the high bar to the low bar. She fractured her cervical vertebra and had surgery.

The remaining two female injuries involved the vault. One happened in a meet, and the circumstances of the second were unknown. Both vaulting injuries were fractures to the spinal column and involved permanent disability.

Table 5.3   Gymnastics Catastrophic Injuries, 1982-1983 to 1991-1992

Year	High school	College	Total
1982-1983	0	0	0
1983-1984	1	1	2
1984-1985	2	0	2
1985-1986	0	1	1
1986-1987	1	0	1
1987-1988	1	0	1
1988-1989	0	0	0
1989-1990	0	0	0
1990-1991	0	0	0
1991-1992	0	0	0
Total	5	2	7

The disability injury rate for high school males was 1.75 per 100,000 participants and for females 1.28 per 100,000 for the period from 1982 to 1992. If males and females are combined, the disability injury rate per 100,000 is 1.35 (Table 5.4).

There were two disability injuries to college gymnasts during this same time period—one to a female and one to a male. The female gymnast fractured a cervical vertebra, but the circumstances of the activity were not available. The male athlete was injured on the high bar and fractured a cervical vertebra during the dismount.

For the 10-year period of this research, the disability injury rate per 100,000 participants was 11.15 for males and 5.92 for females, with a combined rate of 7.73.

Gymnastics Serious Injuries (1982-1992)

In addition to the disability injuries, there were also four serious injuries in gymnastics (Table 5.5). Three were at the high school level and one was at

Table 5.4   High School and College Gymnastics Catastrophic Injuries per 100,000 Participants

Athletes	High school	College
Male	1.75	11.15
Female	1.28	5.92
Combined	1.35	7.73

Table 5.5   Serious Gymnastics Injuries,* 1982-1983 to 1991-1992

Year	High school	College	Total
1982-1983	1	0	1
1983-1984	0	1	1
1984-1985	1	0	1
1985-1986	0	0	0
1986-1987	0	0	0
1987-1988	1	0	1
1988-1989	0	0	0
1989-1990	0	0	0
1990-1991	0	0	0
1991-1992	0	0	0
Total	3	1	4

*Serious injuries are defined as possible disability injuries but with complete recovery.

the college level. The high school injuries all involved injuries to the cervical vertebrae—two fractures and one subluxation injury.

One gymnast received a subluxation of cervical vertebrae 5 and 6 during a tumbling pass (round-off, back handspring, back tuck). She failed to complete the rotation on the last tuck in the last series. There was no permanent disability. Another was injured after a fall off the uneven bars, and the cause of one was unknown. All three of these injuries took place in practice and involved females.

The one college serious injury involved the high bar. The gymnast was injured during the second workout of the day. At the time of the accident, he was performing a dismount from the high bar that involved a foward somersault with 1-1/2 twists. His legs hit the bar and he landed on the mats with his neck fully flexed and his feet hitting the mat behind his head. He had transient paralysis with recovery.

The serious injury rate per 100,000 participants was less than one at the high school level, but the male rate at the college level was 11.15 per 100,000 participants, and the combined rate was 3.87 (Table 5.6).

Table 5.6   High School and College Gymnastics Serious Injuries per 100,000 Participants

Athletes	High school	College
Male	0.00	11.15
Female	0.96	0.00
Combined	0.81	3.87

Swimming

People have been swimming for thousands of years, but the birth of modern competitive swimming is said to have occurred in London in 1837. Competitive swimming at the college level in the United States started in 1897 at the University of Pennsylvania (2). The first meet was between Columbia University, the University of Pennsylvania, and Yale University (3).

In 1982–83, swimming was ranked as the 10th most popular sport for high school males with 76,657 participants in 3,650 schools. In that same year, swimming was the seventh most popular high school female sport with 76,261 participants in 3,497 schools. By 1991–92, the number of male swimmers had increased slightly to 78,474 participants in 4,351 schools; however, there was a much greater increase in female high school swimmers: to 93,545 participants in 4,380 schools. An interesting note is that in 1991–92, swimming was still ranked as the 10th most popular sport for high school males, and it moved to 9th most popular for females.

College participation numbers also show a slight increase in male participation and a greater increase in female participation. In 1982–83, there were 7,427 male participants in 380 colleges and 6,627 females in 361 colleges. In 1991–92, the number of males increased to 7,867, but the number of colleges decreased to 369. In that same 10-year period, the number of females increased to 7,968 and the number of colleges with women's swim programs increased to 391. There is no doubt that Title IX legislation has been responsible for the greater increase in women's programs.

Direct Swimming Fatalities (1982-1992)

For the 10-year period from 1982–83 to 1991–92, the National Center for Catastrophic Sports Injury Research (NCCSIR) did not record any direct fatalities for high school or college swimming programs.

Indirect Swimming Fatalities (1982-1992)

As shown in Table 5.7, there were a total of four indirect fatalities at the high school and college levels for the 10-year period indicated. Three of the fatalities were at the high school level and one at the college level.

All three of the high school indirect fatalities involved females, and the college fatality involved a male. Two of the high school fatalities occurred in practice and the third took place during a meet in a race. The college fatality took place during a preseason run.

Two of the high school deaths involved sudden cardiac death, and the third was related to an asthma attack. One of the cardiac deaths involved a 14-year-old female high school swimmer who died shortly after losing consciousness while swimming laps during practice. Cause of death was unknown, and she

Table 5.7   High School and College Indirect Swimming Fatalities, 1982-1983 to 1991-1992

Year	High school	College	Total
1982-1983	0	0	0
1983-1984	0	0	0
1984-1985	0	0	0
1985-1986	0	0	0
1986-1987	1	0	1
1987-1988	1	1	2
1988-1989	1	0	1
1989-1990	0	0	0
1990-1991	0	0	0
1991-1992	0	0	0
Total	3	1	4

had no known medical history that could account for the death. The case was under litigation.

The college fatality happened during a preseason conditioning run in hot September weather. The athlete suffered heat stroke and died.

As illustrated in Table 5.8, the indirect fatality rate per 100,000 high school participants was less than one, and was only slightly higher at the college level.

Swimming Disability Injuries (1982-1992)

Although catastrophic injuries are usually not associated with swimming, there have been a number of catastrophic injuries recorded with the change in the competitive racing dive. In the early years of swimming competition, the racing dive was a flat dive started from the edge of the pool. The swimmer did not get much depth and started the swim stroke almost immediately. Even when use of the starting blocks began in the 1940s, the racing dive used was the flat dive.

This changed in the 1970s with the change of the flat racing dive to the pike dive. The pike dive, also called the in-the-hole dive or scoop dive, involved the swimmer entering the water at a much steeper angle and getting more depth.

However, the dive itself has not been the problem. The problem has been that the starting blocks in most pools are located in the shallow ends. Using the pike dive into the shallow end of the pool has increased the possibility of the swimmer striking the bottom of the pool with the top or crown of the head, with axial loading to the spinal column.

All of the catastrophic injuries discussed in this chapter have involved the racing start. There have been no competitive diving board accidents recorded at either the high school or college levels since the initiation of this research project.

As shown in Table 5.9 (page 84), there were eight catastrophic or disability injuries at the high school and college levels for the 10-year period under consideration. Seven were at the high school level and one at the college level. All but one of the high school injuries involved trauma to the cervical vertebrae and took place while the swimmer was using the racing dive into the shallow end of the pool.

The one high school injury to the head happened while the athlete was practicing diving onto a port-o-pit (a portable pit filled with foam that can be used away from the pool area). Four of the high school injuries took place in

Table 5.8   High School and College Swimming Indirect Fatalities per 100,000 Participants

Athletes	High school	College
Male	0.00	1.26
Female	0.36	0.00
Combined	0.18	0.64

Table 5.9   Catastrophic Swimming Injuries, 1982-1983 to 1991-1992

Year	High school	College	Total
1982-1983	0	1	1
1983-1984	0	0	0
1984-1985	0	0	0
1985-1986	0	0	0
1986-1987	0	0	0
1987-1988	2	0	2
1988-1989	4	0	4
1989-1990	1	0	1
1990-1991	0	0	0
1991-1992	0	0	0
Total	7	1	8

practice, three were unknown, and the one college injury also took place in practice. Additional information on a sample of the injuries follows:

Case Studies

A female high school athlete was injured while practice diving into a port-o-pit. She was performing a one and one-half back flip when she struck her head on concrete surrounding the pit. She suffered a severe head injury with permanent disability.

A 6 ft 5 in.-tall college swimmer was rendered quadriplegic while practicing racing starts in water that was four ft deep. He was involved in a drill in which the swimmer dives over a rope stretched across the pool about 5 ft from the end. During the dive, he somersaulted and hit the bottom of the pool with the top of his head. The swimmer was practicing the scoop, or pike, dive.

A female high school swimmer sustained a fracture to cervical vertebra 5 during a swim team practice. The team was practicing racing start dives in the shallow end of the pool. She struck the bottom of the pool with her head and was rendered a C-5 quadriplegic.

Table 5.10 illustrates that disability injury rates at the high school level are all less than 1.00 per 100,000 participants. The rate for males was 0.48 and the rate for females was 0.36. The one college injury shows a rate for males of 1.26 per 100,000 participants, and a combined rate for males and females of 0.64.

Swimming Serious Injuries (1982-1992)

There were only three serious injuries in high school and college swimming, as shown in Table 5.11, and all were at the high school level. The serious injuries

Table 5.10   High School and College Swimming Catastrophic Injuries per 100,000 Participants

Athletes	High school	College
Male	0.48	1.26
Female	0.36	0.00
Combined	0.42	0.64

Table 5.11   High School and College Serious Swimming Injuries, 1982-1983 to 1991-1992

Year	High school	College	Total
1982-1983	2	0	2
1983-1984	0	0	0
1984-1985	0	0	0
1985-1986	0	0	0
1986-1987	1	0	1
1987-1988	0	0	0
1988-1989	0	0	0
1989-1990	0	0	0
1990-1991	0	0	0
1991-1992	0	0	0
Total	3	0	3

Table 5.12   High School and College Swimming Serious Injuries per 100,000 Participants

Athletes	High school	College
Male	0.36	0.00
Female	0.00	0.00
Combined	0.18	0.00

all happened the same way as the disability injuries. All three involved fractured cervical vertebrae while the athlete was performing a racing dive into the shallow end of the pool in practice.

These three athletes had full recovery from their injuries. One of the athletes was a 15-year-old high school swimmer who was injured while practicing racing dives into the shallow end of the pool. He fractured and dislocated two cervical vertebrae after hitting the bottom of the pool with the top of his head.

Table 5.12 (page 85) demonstrates that the injury rate per 100,000 participants for serious injuries is 0.36 for males, with a combined rate for males and females of 0.18.

Wrestling

Wrestling is one of the oldest sports in the world, and in fact was part of the Olympic Games as early as 752 BC. There were no weight classes in those days, and it was man against man. It soon became one of the most popular sports because the Greeks considered it the ideal form of physical competition.

Wrestling is still a very popular sport, but the number of participants has declined in the past 10 years both at the high school and college levels. In 1982–83, the number of wrestling participants at the high school level was 254,581 in 8,272 schools. In 1992–93, the number of participants dropped to 222,025, but the number of schools that sponsor wrestling increased to 8,438.

It is also interesting that in 1982–83, there were eight female participants in high school wrestling, and in 1992–93, there were 404 female participants in 404 schools. During the same period, wrestling continued to be ranked as the eighth most popular sport for high school males.

College wrestling is also a very popular sport, and the National Collegiate Wrestling Championships is one of the most successful. Even with this popularity, the decline in the number of participants has been more dramatic at the college level. In 1982–83, there were 8,155 participants in 351 schools. These numbers in 1992–93 have decreased to 6,578 participants in 265 schools. Lack of financing and dropping of wrestling programs and adding women's sports to meet Title IX requirements have played a major role in this decline at the college level.

Direct Wrestling Fatalities (1982-1992)

As shown in Table 5.13, there were two fatalities in high school wrestling for the 10-year period indicated. One of the fatalities occurred when the wrestler hit heads with his opponent during a practice session, received a subdural hematoma, and later died. He was 15 years old.

The second fatality involved a 14-year-old who died on February 25, 1986, from injuries received in a drill during practice on December 19, 1985. The drill involved three participants jumping into the air to get a ball. The injured athlete landed with his back making initial contact with the mat. Cause of death was listed as a pulmonary emboli from blunt impact to the posterior trunk with intervertebral disc hernia and focal necrosis of the spinal cord.

The fatality injury rate for high school wrestling is less than one (0.08) per 100,000 participants for the period from 1982 to 1992 (Table 5.14).

Table 5.13   High School Direct Catastrophic Wrestling Injuries, 1982-1983 to 1991-1992

Year	Fatalities	Disability	Serious
1982-1983	0	2	0
1983-1984	1	1	.1
1984-1985	0	1	2
1985-1986	1	0	2
1986-1987	0	3	0
1987-1988	0	1	1
1988-1989	0	3	2
1989-1990	0	1	0
1990-1991	0	1	0
1991-1992	0	3	1
Total	2	16	9

Table 5.14   High School Wrestling Direct Catastrophic Injuries per 100,000 Participants

Athletes	Fatalities	Disability	Serious
Male	0.08	0.66	0.37
Female	0.00	0.00	0.00
Combined	0.08	0.66	0.37

For this 10-year period there were no direct wrestling fatalities at the college level.

Indirect Wrestling Fatalities (1982-1992)

Ten high school wrestlers died from indirect causes for the time period covered in this research (Table 5.15, page 88). Nine of the fatalities were heart related and the cause of one was a cerebral aneurysm. Eight of the fatalities took place during matches, and two occurred in practice activity.

At the time of the injury, the athletes were engaged in general activity after the match such as practicing take-downs, warm-ups, a pin hold on an opponent, and collapsing. One case involved a 14-year-old who died after collapsing on the mat 33 s into the first period. He was rolling his opponent over into a pinning hold when they went out of bounds. The official blew his whistle to stop action, but the injured athlete was not able to move. CPR was administered, but they were unable to get a pulse.

Table 5.15   High School and College Wrestling Indirect Fatalities, 1982-1983 to 1991-1992

Year	High school	College
1982-1983	0	0
1983-1984	4	0
1984-1985	2	0
1985-1986	2	0
1986-1987	1	0
1987-1988	0	0
1988-1989	0	0
1989-1990	0	0
1990-1991	1	0
1991-1992	0	0
Total	10	0

Table 5.16   High School Wrestling Indirect Fatalities per 100,000 Participants

Athletes	Rate
Male	0.41
Female	0.00
Combined	0.41

The injury rate per 100,000 participants for the 10-year period was 0.41 (Table 5.16). College wrestling was not associated with any indirect fatalities during this time period.

Wrestling Disability Injuries 1982-1992

As illustrated in Table 5.13 (page 87), there were 16 permanent disability injuries in high school wrestling from 1982 through 1992. All 16 involved injuries to cervical vertebrae and were either fractures or dislocations.

A majority of the disability injuries occurred in take-downs with the wrestler's head and neck hitting the mat, and in some cases the opponent's body weight adding force. Eleven of the disability injuries happened in a match situation, four in practice, and one was unknown.

One case involved an 18-year-old high school wrestler who was injured during a match in the 125-lb weight class. The injured athlete tried to "sit out" of a headlock his opponent had on him, fell to the mat headfirst, and was pinned. He injured a cervical vertebra and is now quadriplegic.

A second case involved a 17-year-old who fractured two cervical vertebrae during a match. He was injured while attempting to reverse his opponent and fell to the mat, striking his head above the right eyebrow at the hairline. He bore the weight of his opponent when falling to the mat. He experienced temporary paralysis, and 3 months later walked out of the hospital with the use of a cane. The prognosis was good but there was some disability.

Table 5.14 (page 87) shows that the disability injury rate per 100,000 participants at the high school level was 0.66 from 1982 to 1992.

During this same period of time, there was one permanent disability injury at the college level. A 19-year-old college wrestler was injured during a match and fractured his fifth and sixth cervical vertebrae. He was wrestling in the 118-lb class.

At the time of the accident, both wrestlers were in a standing position. The injured wrestler's opponent was behind him with his arms around his waist. The opponent applied a half nelson, grabbed a leg, and attempted to take the injured wrestler to the mat. The injured wrestler went down and his head was driven into the mat. The injured athlete had permanent paralysis.

The injury rate per 100,000 participants for disability injuries at the college level is 1.30.

Wrestling Serious Injuries (1982-1992)

In addition to the fatalities and disability injuries at the high school level, there were also nine serious injuries in wrestling. Eight of the injuries involved trauma to the cervical vertebra and one to the thoracic vertebra. Seven of the nine injuries took place in matches and six occurred during take-downs.

In one case, a 17-year-old fractured his fourth and fifth cervical vertebrae during a match. He was wrestling in the take-down position, and was taken to the mat by his opponent using an under arm hook, or tie up. The athlete had surgery and has completely recovered from the injury.

The serious injury rate was 0.37 per 100,000 participants. All nine of the athletes had complete recovery. There were no serious injuries at the college level.

Track and Field

Track and field is listed as one sport, although it is really a variety of activities including running, jumping, and throwing. Running events include races from the 100 yd/m dash to the distance runs of from 1 to 2 miles and the hurdle events. Jumping events include the high jump, long jump, triple jump, and the pole vault. The throwing events are the discus, shot put, javelin, and, in some schools and states, the hammer throw.

Accidental injuries can happen in all of these activities, but to date catastrophic injuries have only been associated with the pole vault and the throwing events. Cross country is also associated with track and field and will be covered in a separate section of this chapter.

It is interesting to note that participation levels for both males and females have declined in track and field for the 10-year period from 1982–83 to 1991–92. In 1982–83, male participation numbered 475,229 athletes in 14,414 schools. This participation number ranked third behind high school football and basketball, and the number of schools ranked second behind basketball. Female participation for that same year numbered 355,652 athletes in 13,957 schools. Both of these figures were second to basketball.

In 1991–92, male participation declined to 417,451 athletes, and ranked as the fourth most popular sport behind football, basketball, and baseball. Female participation also declined in 1991–92 to 327,183 athletes in 13,782 schools. Female track and field continued to rank second to basketball in participation.

These figures do not include the 41,448 males and 31,868 females who participated in indoor track at the high school level in 1991–92. These numbers increased from 33,724 males and 15,993 female indoor participants in 1982–83. The number of high school female indoor track athletes doubled in that 10-year period.

College track and field participation figures are also interesting to study. For the same 10-year period previously mentioned, college male participation declined from 18,565 athletes in 587 schools to 18,214 athletes in 580 schools. College male indoor track athletes increased from 14,004 in 435 schools to 15,119 in 476 schools. College female participation in outdoor track increased from 9,785 athletes in 462 schools to 12,246 athletes in 561 schools. Female indoor track increased dramatically, from 6,773 athletes in 280 schools to 12,246 athletes in 561 schools.

At both the high school and college levels and for both males and females, those participating in indoor track are also participating in outdoor track.

Direct Track and Field Fatalities (1982-1992)

For the 10-year period indicated, high school track and field was associated with nine direct fatalities (Table 5.17). Eight of the fatalities involved male participants and one a female. There was almost an even split between meet and practice fatalities, with five occurring in meets and four in practice situations.

As mentioned in the introduction, catastrophic injuries in track and field almost always involve the pole vault and the throwing events, and current data bear this out. Seven of the nine fatalities were associated with the pole vault, and two involved the athlete being struck by a discus.

Pole vaulting accidents all happen the same way: The athlete bounces out of the landing pit and strikes his or her head either on the surrounding hard surface area or on the metal pole plant area, or the athlete misses the mat completely, landing head or neck first on the hard surface. All of the pole vaulting deaths followed these scenarios.

All seven athletes were males. One case involved a 16-year-old high school athlete who bounced out of the pole vaulting pit during a practice session. The pit measured 16 ft by 16 ft. After striking the back edge of the pit, the athlete

Table 5.17   High School Track Direct Catastrophic Injuries, 1982-1983 to 1991-1992

Year	Fatalities	Disability	Serious
1982-1983	3	0	0
1983-1984	0	1	1
1984-1985	1	0	0
1985-1986	0	1	0
1986-1987	1	0	1
1987-1988	0	0	1
1988-1989	0	0	1
1989-1990	1	1	1
1990-1991	2	1	1
1991-1992	1	2	0
Total	9	6	6

flipped over and landed head first on the hard surface surrounding the pit. He crushed the lower portion of his skull and died.

Another case involved an 18-year-old high school pole vaulter who bounced out of the landing pit during a practice session. He was vaulting 12 ft 6 in. at the time. He struck his head on the asphalt surface surrounding the pit, fractured his skull, and died a day later.

In the two fatalities which did not involve pole vaulting, a male athlete was struck in the chest with a discus in practice and died from heart-related injuries, and a 17-year-old female athlete was struck in the back of the head by a thrown discus. She was walking off the field during a meet as it was being cleared due to an approaching thunderstorm. She was walking through the boys' discus competition area when an athlete made a throw. The athlete died from her injuries.

As shown in Table 5.18, the direct fatality rate per 100,000 participants was 0.17 for males, 0.03 for females, and 0.11 for males and females combined.

For this same period, college track and field was associated with one direct death. This fatality involved a male athlete in practice performing in the pole

Table 5.18   High School Track Catastrophic Injuries per 100,000 Participants, 1982-1983 to 1991-1992

Athletes	Fatalities	Disability	Serious
Male	0.17	0.13	0.13
Female	0.03	0.00	0.00
Combined	0.11	0.07	0.07

vault. He bounced out of the pit and struck his head on the hard surface surrounding the pit. The direct fatality rate per 100,000 participants was 0.30 for males and 0.19 for males and females combined.

Indirect Track and Field Fatalities (1982-1992)

As shown in Table 5.19, high school track and field was associated with 13 indirect fatalities from 1982 to 1992. Eleven of the 13 fatalities were to males, and all but two deaths were heart related. One of these latter deaths involved an athlete's aspiration of his own vomitus, and the cause of the second was laryngeal edema, which is very rare, according to the autopsy report.

Seven of the fatalities occurred during meets, four in practice, and information about two was unknown. The athletes were involved in a variety of activities at the time of their collapse. Two cases are as follows:

Case Studies

A 17-year-old track athlete ran a 10K race on a Saturday and complained of being tired after the race. On Monday, he did not go to school because he had flu-like symptoms, and on Tuesday, he passed out at his home. He was taken to the hospital and died 2 hours later. The autopsy revealed congenital heart disease. Additional information revealed that he was on a strict diet, had lost 12 lb in 3 weeks, and had started the diet with a 2-day fast.

An 18-year-old high school athlete collapsed and died during a track meet. He was running the last leg of the 4 x 800 relay. He had run only a few yards before collapsing. The athlete had had a history of passing out in stressful situations, but was given permission to participate by a cardiologist.

**Table 5.19   High School and College Indirect Track Fatalities,
1982-1983 to 1991-1992**

Year	High school	College
1982-1983	3	0
1983-1984	0	0
1984-1985	2	0
1985-1986	1	0
1986-1987	0	1
1987-1988	1	0
1988-1989	1	0
1989-1990	3	0
1990-1991	2	0
1991-1992	0	0
Total	13	1

The indirect fatality rate per 100,000 participants at the high school level is 0.23 for males, 0.06 for females, and 0.16 for males and females combined (Table 5.20).

There was only one indirect fatality at the college level during this period. The athlete, a male, collapsed while running a 1,500 m race in a meet. Cause of death was heart related. The indirect fatality rate per 100,000 participants at the college level is 0.30 for males and 0.19 for males and females combined.

Track and Field Disability Injuries (1982-1992)

Table 5.17 (page 91) shows six permanent disability injuries in high school track and field for the 10-year period from 1982 to 1992. Causes of disability injuries were identical to the causes of fatalities. All six of the injured athletes were males, with three of the injuries occurring in meets and three in practices.

Five of the injuries involved head trauma, and one was a fractured cervical vertebra. Four of the injuries were associated with the pole vault and two with the throwing events. In two of the pole vaulting injuries, the athletes bounced out of the pit onto the hard surfaced runway; in the other two, the athletes struck their heads in the pole plant area.

One of the pole vaulting accidents involved a 14-year-old athlete who was injured while attempting a pole vault in practice. He lost his grip on the pole while in the air and fell head first into the metal pole plant area. He suffered a fractured skull and a subdural hematoma. He returned to school after surgery but suffered speech problems, a personality change, and right side body movement problems.

Another pole vault accident involved a 17-year-old athlete injured while pole vaulting in a track meet. He landed feet first into the pit and was thrown out of it, striking his head on the surrounding asphalt. He suffered a fractured skull and a subdural hematoma. The athlete was in a coma for 6 days and had some residual blindness, but otherwise was functional.

The injuries in the throwing events included one athlete being struck by a discus and the second being struck by a thrown javelin. The athlete struck by the javelin was 15 years old. He was hit above the right ear. The accident took place in practice, and apparently the javelin was thrown off course by a strong wind. The athlete suffered paralysis to the left side of his body. Permanent

Table 5.20   High School and College Track Indirect Fatality Rate per 100,000 Participants, 1982-1983 to 1991-1992

Athletes	High school	College
Male	0.23	0.30
Female	0.06	0.00
Combined	0.16	0.19

disability injury rates per 100,000 participants were 0.13 for males and 0.07 for males and females combined (Table 5.18, page 91).

College track and field was associated with three permanent disability injuries during this time period. One athlete was injured in the pole vault during a meet, and two athletes were struck by the hammer—one in practice and one in a meet. All three of the athletes were males, and all suffered head injuries.

One of the athletes, 23 years old, was injured after being struck in the head by an errant 16-lb metal ball (hammer throw). He suffered a serious head injury and was in a coma for 3 weeks. The athlete was involved in rehabilitation, and recovery was incomplete. The permanent disability rate per 100,000 participants was 0.90 for males and 0.56 for males and females combined.

Serious Track and Field Injuries (1982-1992)

In addition to the track and field fatalities and permanent disability injuries, there were six serious injuries at the high school level (Table 5.17, page 91). All of the injuries were to males, with four injuries taking place in practice sessions and two in meets. Three of the injured athletes were participating in the pole vault, one was struck with a discus, one was struck by a shot put, and one was injured by a javelin. Four of the injuries involved head trauma, one an injury to a thoracic vertebra, and one a puncture wound to the stomach.

One of the athletes was a 16-year-old high school discus thrower. He was struck in the head by a discus thrown by another member of the team. The injured athlete was standing outside the discus circle when he was struck. He received a fractured skull but had a full recovery with no disability. Table 5.18 (page 91) shows the serious injury rate per 100,000 participants was 0.13 for males and 0.07 for males and females combined.

Cheerleading

Cheerleading has its roots in the competitive atmosphere of sporting events and began around the same time as American football, with young men leading the cheers and school songs at sporting events. According to A.B. Frederick, cheerleading has gone through three distinct periods (4).

In the pre-World War II era, cheerleading was a student-organized activity that consisted of yelling cheers and simple tumbling. After World War II, cheerleading spread rapidly across the country, and equipment like the miniature trampoline began to be used in gymnastics maneuvers, which increased the possibility of accidents. During the last period, from approximately 1975 to the present, the number of participants has grown to hundreds of thousands, stunts have become increasingly complex, competitions have been organized for a national championship, and summer training camps have become popular.

The Consumer Product Safety Commission reported an estimated 4,954 hospital emergency room visits in 1980 caused by cheerleading injuries. By 1986, that number increased to 6,911, and has continued to grow. The NCCSIR began collecting cheerleading catastrophic injury data when a number of cases were reported at the college level in 1982-83.

Cheerleading is not usually considered a sport, and therefore reliable participation numbers are not available. However, a rough estimate of high school and college cheerleaders would be 250,000 participants per year at the high school level and 10,000 at the college level.

Direct Cheerleading Fatalities (1982-1992)

There were two direct cheerleading fatalities during the 10-year period from 1982 to 1992. High school and college cheerleading each accounted for one (as shown in Tables 5.21 and 5.22). The high school cheerleader was injured and died a week after the accident. She fell from a double level cheerleading stance during practice and struck her head on the gym floor, suffering massive head injuries.

The college cheerleader also died from injuries suffered during a cheerleading stunt. Her injuries included multiple skull fractures and massive brain damage. The athlete fell from the top level of a pyramid stunt and struck her head on the gym floor. She died a week after the accident. The direct fatality injury rate, if one used the estimates provided, would be 0.04 per 100,000 participants at the high school level and 1.00 per 100,000 participants at the college level.

Disability Injuries in Cheerleading (1982-1992)

There were five permanent disability injuries at the high school level for the 10-year period previously mentioned. A majority of these injuries happen when the athlete falls from a pyramid stunt or is dropped during a basket catch or during another activity that involves being caught during a cheerleading stunt. Following are the cases involving high school cheerleading disability injuries:

Table 5.21   High School Cheerleading Direct Catastrophic Injuries, 1982-1983 to 1991-1992

Year	Fatalities	Disability	Serious
1982-1983	0	0	0
1983-1984	0	0	0
1984-1985	0	1	0
1985-1986	0	1	0
1986-1987	0	0	0
1987-1988	0	2	1
1988-1989	0	0	1
1989-1990	0	1	1
1990-1991	0	0	1
1991-1992	1	0	0
Total	1	5	4

**Table 5.22   College Cheerleading Direct Catastrophic Injuries,
1982-1983 to 1991-1992**

Year	Fatalities	Disability	Serious
1982-1983	0	1	1
1983-1984	0	0	2
1984-1985	0	1	0
1985-1986	1	1	0
1986-1987	0	0	1
1987-1988	0	0	0
1988-1989	0	0	0
1989-1990	0	0	1
1990-1991	0	0	0
1991-1992	0	0	1
Total	1	3	6

Case Studies

A high school cheerleader was injured during a practice session after falling from the top level of a pyramid. She struck her head and neck on a hard surface and was partially paralyzed.

A high school cheerleader was attempting to complete a back flip off the shoulders of another cheerleader. She landed on her head and neck, fractured a cervical vertebra, and was diagnosed as quadriplegic.

A high school cheerleader fell from a pyramid in practice. She was 6 ft off the floor when she fell, and was not using spotters. Her injuries included a fractured collarbone, a damaged ear drum, and a basal skull fracture. She has suffered a partial hearing loss and must wear special glasses for reading.

A high school cheerleader was tossed into the air by two of her teammates and was supposed to flip backward and land feet first on the shoulders of two other cheerleaders. She fell on a hard surface during the stunt and was paralyzed from the waist down.

A high school cheerleader fractured a cervical vertebra during practice. She was performing a series of back flips during a tumbling run, slipped on the wet grass, and landed on her neck. She is now quadriplegic.

The disability injury rate for high school cheerleaders was 0.2 per 100,000 participants. This rate is very low, but many believe that there should not be any catastrophic injuries in cheerleading.

Disability injuries at the college level numbered three from 1982 to 1992. The etiology of college injuries is no different from that of the high school injuries. A cheerleader falls from a pyramid stunt and strikes a hard surface or is dropped during another stunt. Following are the cases involving college disability injuries:

Case Studies

A cheerleader was injured after diving from a mini-trampoline over several cheerleaders while cheering at a basketball game. The stunt was called a dive into a forward roll. He fractured and dislocated several cervical vertebrae and had permanent paralysis.

A college cheerleader fractured her skull in practice after falling from the top level of a three high pyramid. She struck her head on the wood floor in the gym. She was in critical condition for a period of time, but was released from the hospital and is now involved in occupational therapy. She has permanent disabilities.

A cheerleader was paralyzed after a fall in practice. He was attempting a front flip from a mini-trampoline. He dislocated several cervical vertebrae and is now quadriplegic.

The disability injury rate at the college level was 3.0 per 100,000 participants. When compared with other college sports, this rate is fairly high.

Serious Injuries in Cheerleading (1982-1992)

From 1982 through 1992 there were four high school serious cheerleading injuries (Table 5.21, page 95). The etiology is exactly the same as in the disability injuries, and in most cases can be prevented. The serious injury rate is 0.2 per 100,000 participants in high school cheerleading.

As shown in Table 5.22 (page 96), there were six serious injuries in college cheerleading during this same time period. The case of the college cheerleader who suffered a head injury during practice is a good example of how many of the serious injuries could have been disability injuries or fatalities if there had not been proper medical care or medical facilities.

She was thrown into the air but was not caught by her teammates, and struck her head on the gym floor. She was in critical condition, was upgraded to serious, and is expected to recover. The serious injury rate was 6.0 per 100,000 participants for college cheerleading, a high rate when compared with other college sports.

References

1. Johnson KM: Where have all the gymnasts gone? *J Phys Ed, Rec and Dance.* March 1985.
2. Oppenhein F: *The history of swimming.* N. Hollywood, CA: Swimming World; 1970.
3. Rice EA, et al: *A brief history of physical education.* New York: The Ronald Press Co.; 1958.
4. Frederick AB: Educational and safety materials for cheerleading. *AACCA cheerleading safety manual.* Memphis, TN: UCA Publications; 1990.

Chapter 6

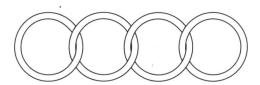

Recommendations for Prevention

The incidence of catastrophic injuries in sports at the high school and college levels is low, but even one is too many. Permanent paralysis, brain damage, and death should not be associated with teenagers and young adults participating in high school and college athletics. Catastrophic injury is devastating not only to the injured athlete, but also to the athlete's family, school, and community.

With proper medical care and safety precautions, a number of these injuries can be prevented. As demonstrated in the chapter on football (chapter 3), it is possible to reduce the number of catastrophic injuries with a good data collection system, the implementation of game rules, proper medical care, and good coaching.

Tables 6.1 through 6.6 (pages 100-102) illustrate that there are some sports with a higher incidence of catastrophic injury than others, but there are also some sports with higher injury rates per 100,000 participants. For example, football has the greatest number of catastrophic injuries, but it also has the greatest number of participants at both levels of play. Gymnastics, ice hockey, and cheerleading have higher rates than football in some categories. Table 6.7 (page 103) gives the participation numbers for high school and college sports for the fall of 1982 through the spring of 1992.

Emphasis should be placed on the fact that no matter how low the incidence levels or rates per number of participants, an increased effort should be placed on prevention and the possible elimination of catastrophic injuries.

Prevention Recommendations for All Sports

The purpose of this section is to make general recommendations for all sports to reduce the number of catastrophic injuries in high school and college athletics.

Table 6.1   Comparison of High School Direct Fatalities by Sport, 1982-1983 to 1991-1992

Sport	Fatalities	Injury rate per 100,000	
		Men	Women
Fall sports			
Football	48	0.35	0.00
Soccer	2	0.10	0.00
Cheerleading	1	Combined 0.04	
Winter sports			
Basketball	0	0.00	0.00
Gymnastics	1	1.75	0.00
Ice hockey	1	0.43	0.00
Swimming	0	0.00	0.00
Wrestling	2	0.08	0.00
Spring sports			
Baseball	3	0.07	0.00
Lacrosse	1	0.57	0.00
Track and field	9	0.17	0.03

Table 6.2   Comparison of High School Disability Injuries by Sport, 1982-1983 to 1991-1992

Sport	Injuries	Injury rate per 100,000	
		Men	Women
Fall sports			
Football	103	0.75	0.00
Soccer	0	0.00	0.00
Cheerleading	5	Combined 2.00	
Winter sports			
Basketball	2	0.02	0.03
Gymnastics	5	1.75	1.28
Ice hockey	4	1.73	0.00
Swimming	4	0.24	0.24
Wrestling	16	0.66	0.00
Spring sports			
Baseball	7	0.17	0.00
Lacrosse	0	0.00	0.00
Track and field	6	0.13	0.00

Table 6.3   Comparison of High School Serious Injuries by Sport, 1982-1983 to 1991-1992

		Injury rate per 100,000	
Sport	Injuries	Men	Women
Fall sports			
Football	112	0.81	0.00
Soccer	4	0.20	0.00
Cheerleading	4	Combined 1.60	
Winter sports			
Basketball	2	0.04	0.00
Gymnastics	3	0.00	0.96
Ice hockey	2	0.86	0.00
Swimming	3	0.36	0.00
Wrestling	9	0.37	0.00
Spring sports			
Baseball	6	0.15	0.00
Lacrosse	0	0.00	0.00
Track and field	6	0.13	0.00

Table 6.4   Comparison of College Direct Fatalities by Sport, 1982-1983 to 1991-1992

		Injury rate per 100,000	
Sport	Fatalities	Men	Women
Fall sports			
Football	3	0.40	0.00
Soccer	0	0.00	0.00
Cheerleading	1	Combined 1.00	
Winter sports			
Basketball	0	0.00	0.00
Gymnastics	0	0.00	0.00
Ice hockey	0	0.00	0.00
Swimming	0	0.00	0.00
Wrestling	0	0.00	0.00
Spring sports			
Baseball	2	0.98	0.00
Lacrosse	0	0.00	0.00
Track and field	1	0.30	0.00

Table 6.5   Comparison of College Disability Injuries by Sport, 1982-1983 to 1991-1992

		Injury rate per 100,000	
Sport	Injuries	Men	Women
Fall sports			
Football	15	2.00	0.00
Soccer	0	0.00	0.00
Cheerleading	3	Combined 3.00	
Winter sports			
Basketball	0	0.00	0.00
Gymnastics	2	11.15	5.92
Ice hockey	1	2.48	0.00
Swimming	1	1.26	0.00
Wrestling	1	1.31	0.00
Spring sports			
Baseball	0	0.00	0.00
Lacrosse	2	2.05	3.35
Track and field	2	0.60	0.00

Table 6.6   Comparison of College Serious Injuries by Sport, 1982-1983 to 1991-1992

		Injury rate per 100,000	
Sport	Injuries	Men	Women
Fall sports			
Football	45	6.00	0.00
Soccer	1	0.70	0.00
Cheerleading	6	Combined 6.00	
Winter sports			
Basketball	2	1.56	0.00
Gymnastics	1	11.15	0.00
Ice hockey	3	7.45	0.00
Swimming	0	0.00	0.00
Wrestling	0	0.00	0.00
Spring sports			
Baseball	1	0.49	0.00
Lacrosse	1	2.05	0.00
Track and field	2	0.60	0.00

Table 6.7   High School and College Participation Numbers, 1982-1983 to 1991-1992

Sport	High school		College	
	Men	Women	Men	Women
Fall sports				
Football	13,800,000	342	750,000	
Soccer	2,021,665	948,161	143,976	51,676
Cheerleading	Combined 250,000		Combined 10,000	
Winter sports				
Basketball	5,113,733	3,907,964	128,018	106,129
Gymnastics	57,062	313,544	8,972	16,891
Ice hockey	231,685	579	40,262	1,324
Swimming	834,029	829,828	79,374	76,109
Wrestling	2,430,450	737	76,398	
Spring sports				
Baseball	4,072,405	4,926	203,925	
Lacrosse	174,506	81,002	48,900	29,861
Track and field	4,712,302	3,578,939	334,560	199,822

Preparticipation Exams

1. Mandatory medical examinations and medical history should be taken before an athlete is allowed to participate. The National Collegiate Athletic Association (NCAA) recommends a thorough medical examination when the athlete first enters the college athletic program and an annual health history update with the use of referral exams when warranted (1). This initial evaluation should include a comprehensive health history, immunization history as defined by the current Center for Disease Control (CDC) guidelines, and a relevant physical exam, part of which should include an orthopedic evaluation.

2. High schools should follow the recommendations set by their state high school athletic associations. If there are no set recommendations, the NCAA guidelines are appropriate.

3. If the physician or coach has any questions about the readiness of the athlete, the athlete should not be allowed to participate.

4. Recommendations concerning sudden death in athletes made by Dr. Van Camp in chapter 2 should be followed.

Proper Conditioning

1. All personnel concerned with training athletes should emphasize proper, gradual, and complete physical conditioning. Adequate conditioning includes cardiovascular conditioning and development of muscular strength and flexibility.

2. An important area of muscular strength development is the muscles of the neck. Neck muscles should be strengthened and players educated concerning risk of neck injuries.

Medical Care

1. Medical coverage of both practice and game situations is important. Certified athletic trainers can provide good medical coverage, but a physician should be on call for practices and possibly present at games. More than half of the catastrophic injuries occur in games, and a physician on-site would be advantageous. Written emergency procedures should be prepared in advance.

2. An athlete who has experienced or shown signs of head trauma (loss of consciousness, visual disturbances, headache, inability to walk correctly, obvious disorientation, memory loss) should receive immediate medical attention and should not be allowed to play, practice, or cheer without permission from the proper medical authorities.

3. Emergency plans in case of a catastrophic injury should be written and distributed to all personnel involved with the program. Personnel will include, but not be limited to, the head coach, assistant coaches, managers, athletic trainers, and physicians. Players should also be made aware of emergency procedures. If everyone understands his or her responsibility in the event of a catastrophic injury, the chances of permanent disability may be reduced.

4. Each institution should strive to have a team trainer who is a regular member of the faculty and is adequately prepared and qualified. Trainers certified by the National Athletic Trainers Association (NATA) are preferred.

5. Coaches should never be involved in making medical decisions concerning athletes, and only medical personnel should decide if and when an athlete returns to play after an injury or illness.

6. Cooperation should be maintained by all groups interested in the field of athletic medicine (coaches, trainers, physicians, manufacturers, administrators).

Heat Illness

According to the American Academy of Pediatrics Committee on Sports Medicine, heat-related illnesses are all preventable (2). The following practices and precautions are recommended:

1. All personnel associated with athletic participation should understand the proper safety measures for activity in hot weather.

2. Each athlete should have a complete physical examination with medical history and an annual health history update. History of previous heat illness and type of training activities prior to organized practice should be included.

3. Lack of physical fitness impairs the performance of athletes who participate in high temperatures. Coaches should know the physical condition of athletes and set practice schedules accordingly.

4. Along with physical conditioning, the factor of acclimatization to heat is important. Acclimatization is the process of becoming adjusted to heat, and *gradual* acclimatization to hot weather is essential. Athletes must exercise in the heat if they are to become acclimatized to it. It is suggested that a gradual physical conditioning program be used, and that 80% acclimatization can be expected to occur after the first 7 to 10 days. Final stages of acclimatization to heat are marked by increased sweating and reduced salt concentration in the sweat.

5. Knowledge of both the temperature and the humidity is important, since it is more difficult for the body to cool itself in high humidity. Use of a sling psychrometer is recommended to measure the relative humidity: Anytime the wet-bulb temperature is over 78°, practice should be altered.

6. It is important to adjust activity level and provide frequent rest periods. Athletes should rest in cool shaded areas with some air movement, and remove helmets and loosen or remove jerseys. Rest periods totaling 15 to 30 min should be provided during workouts of 1 hr.

7. Adequate cold water replacement during practice should be provided. Water should always be available to the athlete in unlimited quantities. *WATER SHOULD BE GIVEN REGULARLY.*

8. Salt should be replaced daily, and liberal salting of the athletes' food will accomplish this purpose. Coaches should not provide salt tablets to athletes. Attention must be directed to water replacement.

9. Athletes should weigh in each day before and after practice and weight charts should be checked in order to treat the athlete who loses excessive weight each day. Generally, a 3% body weight loss through sweating is safe, and a 5% loss is in the danger zone.

10. Clothing is important, and a player should avoid use of long stockings and excess clothing. Athletes should never use rubberized clothing or sweat suits.

11. Some athletes are more susceptible to heat injury. These individuals are not accustomed to working in the heat, may be overweight, and may be those eager athletes who constantly compete at their capacity. Athletes with previous heat problems should be watched closely.

12. It is important to observe for signs of heat illness. Some trouble signs are nausea, incoherence, fatigue, weakness, vomiting, cramps, weak rapid pulse, flushed appearance, visual disturbance, and unsteadiness. If heat illness is suspected, seek a physician's immediate service. Recommended emergency procedures are vital.

13. An increased number of medical personnel are now treating heat illness by applying either alcohol or cool water to the victim's skin and then fanning vigorously. The fanning causes evaporation and cooling. This can be done by the coach or athletic trainer while waiting for medical assistance or an ambulance.

Proper Training of Coaches

1. It is imperative to hire coaches with the ability and expertise to teach the proper fundamental skills of the game.

2. Competent coaching in athletics is a major area of concern. High schools are having a difficult time employing coaches who are full time faculty members, and in many cases have to hire part time coaches. This is not a problem if these coaches know the fundamental skills of the sport and have the ability to teach these skills to the participants. Improper teaching of sport skills can be a direct cause of injuries—both catastrophic and others.

3. In some sports, coaching certifications are available. Coaches in these sports should be certified. In addition, a small number of states require that their high school coaches have a coaching certification. This is a step in the right direction, and should receive increased emphasis.

4. Coaches should keep up to date with new safety procedures and safety equipment.

5. There should be an emphasis on providing excellent facilities, and securing the safest and best equipment possible.

Supporting Referees' Decisions

1. There should be strict enforcement of game rules, and administrative regulations should be enforced to protect the health of the athlete. Coaches and school officials must support the game officials in their decisions during sports events. Strict enforcement of the rules of the game by both coaches and officials will help reduce serious injuries.

2. Officiating is also important when discussing injury prevention. Quality officials can spot dangerous situations during a game or match, and can stop the activity before it results in a serious or catastrophic injury.

Sport-Specific Recommendations

Football

1. Rule changes initiated for the 1976 football season that eliminated the use of the head and face as the initial contact area for blocking and tackling are of the utmost importance. Coaches should continue to emphasize and teach the proper fundamentals of blocking and tackling to help reduce catastrophic head and neck injuries. Both present and past data show that poorly executed tackling and blocking is the major cause of cervical spine injuries, not the football helmet. *SHOULDER BLOCK AND TACKLE WITH THE HEAD UP—KEEP THE HEAD OUT OF FOOTBALL.*

2. The use of the helmet-face mask in making initial contact is illegal, and should be called for a penalty. If more of these penalties are called, there is no doubt that both coaches and players will get the message and discontinue this type of play.

3. There should be continued research concerning the safety factor in football (rules, facilities, equipment, etc.).

4. Players should be taught to respect the football helmet as a protective device, and that it should not be used as a weapon.

5. Coaches, trainers, and physicians should take special care to see that the players' equipment is properly fitted, particularly the helmet.

Soccer

The main problem in soccer catastrophic injuries has been soccer goals falling on the participants, or children climbing on the goals. The most recent case occurred in June 1992 when a steel frame soccer goal fell on and crushed the skull of a 6-year-old boy. The injury resulted in death. A Loss Control Bulletin from K & K Insurance Group, Inc., of Fort Wayne, IN, suggests the following safeguards (3):

1. Keep soccer goals supervised and anchored.

2. Never permit hanging or climbing on a soccer goal.

3. Always stand to the rear or side of the goal when moving it—NEVER to the front.

4. Stabilize the goal as best suits the playing surface, but in a manner that does not create other hazards to players.

5. Develop and follow a plan for periodic inspection and maintenance (e.g., dry rot, joints, hooks).

6. Advise all field maintenance persons to re-anchor the goal if moved for mowing the grass or other purposes.

7. Remove goals from fields no longer in use for the soccer program as the season progresses.

8. Secure goals well from unauthorized access when stored.

9. Educate and remind all players and adult supervisors about the past tragedies of soccer goal fatalities.

Basketball

Direct fatalities and catastrophic injuries at both the high school and college levels are minimal. This means that the injuries should continue to be monitored and that the present rules and safety measures should be enforced.

In basketball, the problem is indirect fatalities—37 at the high school level and 8 at the college level. This is an area where continued surveillance is important, and emphasis should be placed on the preseason medical examination.

Ice Hockey

Ice hockey injuries are low in number, but the injury rates per 100,000 participants are high when compared with other sports, both at the high school and college levels (Tables 6.1-6.6, pages 100-102). Ice hockey catastrophic injuries usually occur when the athlete is struck from behind by an opponent, slides head first into the boards surrounding the rink, and makes contact with the top or crown of the head. The results are usually a fractured cervical vertebra with paralysis.

Research in Canada has revealed high catastrophic injury rates with similar results. After an in-depth study of ice hockey catastrophic injuries in Canada, Dr. Charles Tator has made the following recommendations concerning prevention (4):

1. Enforce current rules and consider new rules against pushing or checking from behind.

2. Continue epidemiological research in injury data collection, equipment, and rink construction.

3. Educate players concerning the risk of neck injuries related to rule violations.

Baseball

Catastrophic injuries in high school and college baseball usually happen in one of the following three ways:

1. The athlete is hit by either a thrown or batted ball, resulting in a serious head injury or a chest impact death.

2. The athlete collides with a teammate while chasing a fly ball, resulting in a serious head or neck injury. Collisions usually involve an infielder and an outfielder or two outfielders chasing the same fly ball.

3. The athlete uses the head first slide and makes contact with the top or crown of the head and the opposing player's lower body or the base. This type of injury usually results in a fractured cervical vertebra with possible paralysis.

As illustrated in Tables 6.1 to 6.6 (pages 100-102), baseball catastrophic injuries do not happen very frequently, and the catastrophic injury rate per 100,000 participants is low for both high school and college programs. Proper preventive measures can be implemented to further reduce the chance of catastrophic injuries in baseball. These preventive measures are as follows:

1. Coaches should teach the proper skills of the head first slide if it is going to be used. Players should be warned that, if not properly executed, the head first slide can result in serious or disability injuries.

2. It should be made mandatory for all players to wear batting helmets in practice as well as in game situations. Batting practice pitchers should wear protective helmets. Coaches should be no exception. Proper fitting of the helmets should be stressed.

3. Student managers and nonplayers should be required to wear protective helmets when on the field.

4. Protective screens should be used to protect the batting practice pitchers and other players who may be involved in other activities during batting practice. Coaches should be no exception.

5. Strategies that can and should be used when two players from the same team are chasing a fly ball should be discussed and taught.

Lacrosse

Lacrosse has not been associated with a great number of catastrophic injuries over the years, but the participation figures are low at both the high school and college levels, which makes the injury rate higher in lacrosse when compared with other sports. This is especially true at the college level. To keep the number of catastrophic injuries low, the following is recommended:

1. Injury research at both the high school and college levels is essential. At the present time there is a lack of good injury research in lacrosse.

2. Current rules which make it illegal to use the head in contact should be enforced.

3. Research in the type of equipment that is mandatory for lacrosse players should be continued.

4. Coaching certification for coaches is important in a sport like lacrosse that involves many skills and body contact.

5. Women's lacrosse is changing rapidly and in some instances is influenced by the men's game. Decisions on rule and equipment changes should be based on safety concerns and the results of adequate injury data.

Gymnastics

It is important to mention that with such a small number of catastrophic injuries in gymnastics, it is difficult to make safety recommendations based on the data. However, as in all sports, there are safety recommendations that should be followed. The United States Gymnastics Federation recommends the following safety guidelines (5):

1. Athletes should be made aware of the risks involved in gymnastics, and that there is the possibility of catastrophic injury, paralysis, and death.

2. Competent supervision—a gymnast should never participate in gymnastics activity without competent supervision.

3. Be prepared to participate—dress appropriately, follow accepted warm-up practices, and be mentally prepared to engage in activity.

4. Carefully check equipment—before activity make sure the equipment is adjusted and secured properly and that adequate matting appropriate to the activity is in the correct position.

5. Carelessness cannot be tolerated—gymnastics is an activity requiring active concentration. Horseplay or any form of carelessness cannot be tolerated at any time for any reason.

6. Follow proper skill progressions—a safe learning environment includes a correct understanding of the skill being performed and following proper skill progressions.

7. Mastering basic skills—safe learning practices demand mastering basic skills before progressing to new or more difficult skills.

8. Attempting new or difficult skills—the readiness and ability level of the performer, the nature of the task, and the competency of the spotter all must be taken into consideration when attempting a new or difficult skill.

9. Proper landing technique—safe dismounts, as well as unintentional falls, require proper landing techniques. No amount of matting can be fail-safe. Avoid landing on head or neck at all costs, as serious catastrophic injuries may result.

Swimming

A recent advertisement from a company that manufactures starting blocks also included a warning notice. This notice stated that since the development of the pike dive, competitive swimmers have sustained serious cervical injuries resulting in quadriplegia. It continues by strongly recommending that starting blocks not be used for deep entry into the water until the pool depth has been determined.

It is apparent that, because all of the catastrophic injuries follow the same etiology, the recommendations for prevention will focus on the racing dive.

1. If possible, the starting blocks should be moved to the deep end of the pool.

2. The proper fundamental skills needed for a successful dive must be taught if the pike dive is to be used as a racing start.

3. Swimmers must be warned concerning the possibility of catastrophic injury when using the pike dive in the shallow end of the pool.

4. All involved should be knowledgeable concerning the National Federation of State High School Associations (NFSHSA) rules governing the racing dive and water depth. These rules state that in 4 or more feet of water, the swimmers may use a starting platform up to a maximum of 30 in. above the water. With a water depth of between 3-1/2 and 4 ft, swimmers may start no higher than 18 in. above the water. With less than 3-1/2 ft of water, the swimmers must start the race in the pool. These rules are being monitored, and a research project concerning a safe pool depth for the pike dive is in progress.

5. A plan should be developed to be prepared for a catastrophic injury situation. All staff members and swimmers should be aware of this plan and of their role in carrying out their duties.

Wrestling

All of the wrestling catastrophic injuries, with the exception of one college disability injury, took place at the high school level. When discussing prevention of wrestling injuries, it is important to emphasize a few key areas:

1. Proper supervision at both practice and matches is important. Any activity that is potentially dangerous should be stopped immediately.

2. Good quality mats and knowledge of how they are set up for both practices and matches is crucial.

3. Competent coaching in a sport like wrestling is a major area of concern. Improper teaching of the skills of wrestling can be the direct cause of catastrophic injuries.

4. Quality officials can spot dangerous holds and can stop the activity before it results in a serious or catastrophic injury.

Track and Field

The pole vault has been associated with the majority of catastrophic track injuries, while injuries from being hit during the throwing events ranked second. There is no excuse for someone being hit with a shot put, discus, hammer, or javelin. All of these injuries are preventable.

The NFSHSA Track and Field Rules Committee adopted three rule changes for the pole vault that will go into effect in the 1995 season. Rule 7-4-3 states that the vaulter's weight shall be at or below the manufacturer's pole rating, and that the manufacturer's pole rating shall be visible in a 1 in. contrasting color. A vaulter using an illegal pole shall be immediately disqualified from the event.

Rule 7-4-15 allows the crossbar to be moved a maximum of 30 in. in the direction of the landing surface. The previous rule limited the distance to 24 in. This change will allow the bar to be moved deeper in the landing pad, which will allow vaulters to penetrate further back on the landing mat.

Rule 7-4-7 recommends that concrete, metal, wood, or asphalt surfaces that extend out from under the landing pad be cut away and removed. If this is not possible, these hard surfaces should be padded with a minimum of 2 in. of dense foam or other suitable material.

The NFSHSA also recommended the following safety recommendations for the pole vault:

1. Landing pads should be maintained, reconditioned, or replaced if they lose their density or load capabilities.

2. Proper supervision should be provided at all times. A vaulter should not be allowed to vault alone.

3. By rule, all exposed projections on the base of the standards or uprights must be padded or covered. Adjustment knobs should be located on the outside of the standards.

4. By rule, the base of the standards must be anchored to minimize the possibility of a displaced crossbar or released vaulting pole knocking a standard into the landing pit.

5. Only a non-metal, circular crossbar be used.

6. Vaulting poles should be constantly inspected for cracks or dents that can reduce the original stress level of the pole.

7. Special clinics emphasizing safety procedures and appropriate teaching techniques should be offered for coaches who do not have a strong background in vaulting.

8. Pole vaulters need a significant amount of diversified conditioning before they are allowed to vault for height.

9. Coaches should emphasize how the vaulter arrives at the decision to abort a vault that may or may not get into the landing pad.

10. The first rule for terminating an attempt after becoming airborne is to hang onto the pole and look for a safe place to land, then release the pole if over the landing pad, or ride the pole to the safest landing area.

11. If smaller or minimum landing pads are in use, caution should be urged where 14-ft poles or less are used.

12. The space between the stop-board and landing pad should be covered by wrestling mat material or similar padded material.

13. Correct alignment and safe pole penetration is urged at all times.

14. With a large bend and deep penetration, a stronger pole should be used. With a small bend and deep penetration, a higher grip, not to exceed limitations, should be used. With a large bend and poor penetration, a lower grip should be used. With a small bend and poor penetration, a softer pole, not below the body weight, should be used. (A large bend would be defined as 90° or more.)

Safety precautions for the throwing events must be stressed in both practice and competitive meets. All of these accidents are preventable. The 1993 rule that fences off the back and sides of the discus circle should help. Good risk management and supervision should also be implemented.

Cheerleading

1. Cheerleaders should be trained by a qualified coach with training in gymnastics. This person should also be trained in the proper methods for spotting and other safety procedures.

2. Cheerleaders should receive proper training and instruction before attempting gymnastic-type stunts, and should not attempt stunts they are not capable of completing. A qualification system demonstrating mastery of stunts in progression is recommended.

3. Coaches should supervise all practice sessions in a safe facility.

4. Mini-trampolines and flips off pyramids and shoulders should be prohibited.

5. Pyramid and partner stunts over shoulder level should not be performed without mats and spotters.

6. There should be continued research concerning safety in cheerleading.

7. There is no excuse for the number of participants being injured. Cheerleading should be conducted within the limits of safety. The American Association of Cheerleading Coaches and Advisors Safety Certification Program has been implemented and over 500 coaches have participated in safety certification programs.

According to the NFSHSA, the primary purpose of spirit groups (cheerleaders) is to serve as support groups for the interscholastic athletic programs within the school. In January of 1993, 18 rule revisions were adopted for spirit groups. One of the major rules prohibits tumbling over, under, or through people or equipment. All of the rules were adopted to enhance the safety of the participants. Copies of spirit group rules are available from the NFSHSA.

References

1. National Collegiate Athletic Association. *1993-94 NCAA sports medicine handbook.* 6th ed. Overland Park, KS; 1993.
2. American Academy of Pediatrics. *Sports medicine: health care for young athletes.* 2nd ed. Elk Grove Village, IL; 1991.
3. K&K Insurance Group, Inc. *Loss Control Bulletin, Soccer Injuries.* Fort Wayne, IN; 1993.
4. Tator CH, et al: National survey of spinal injuries in hockey players. *Can Med Assoc J.* April 1, 1984; 30.
5. George GS. *USGF gymnastics safety manual.* Indianapolis: The USGF Publications Dept.; 1985.

About the Authors

Frederick O. Mueller is director of the National Center for Catastrophic Sports Injury Research located at the University of North Carolina at Chapel Hill. Mueller has been active since 1968 in research on athletic injury, and his contributions have helped to significantly reduce the number of football fatalities and paralyzing injuries and to make sports safer for all participants.

Mueller has written more than 75 articles on sport safety, edited *Prevention of Athletic Injuries*—a book on sports medicine and injury reduction, and presented his findings at national and international sport safety meetings. Mueller, who earned a PhD in Education/Physical Education in 1970 from the University of North Carolina at Chapel Hill, is a member of the American College of Sports Medicine (ACSM), the American Football Coaches Association, and the American Alliance for Health, Physical Education, Recreation and Dance (AAHPERD).

Robert C. Cantu, MD, is past president of the American College of Sports Medicine and medical director of the National Center for Catastrophic Sports Injury Research. He has authored more than 180 scientific works, including 14 books on neurology and sports medicine, numerous book chapters, scholarly articles, and video programs. He is an associate editor of *Medicine and Science in Sports and Exercise* and *Exercise and Sports Science Reviews* and serves on the editorial boards of *The Physician and Sportsmedicine* and *Clinical Journal of Sports Medicine*.

Cantu earned a master's degree in endocrinology in 1962 and an MD in 1963 from the University of California Medical School in San Francisco. A member of more than 25 professional organizations, including ACSM and the American Association of Neurological Surgeons, he is vice president of the National Operating Committee for Standards for Athletic Equipment (NOCSAE).

Cantu serves as chief neurosurgeon and director of sports medicine at Emerson Hospital in Concord, Massachusetts.

Steven P. Van Camp, MD, president of the ACSM, is a cardiologist in private practice in San Diego and medical director of both the Alvarado Hospital Medical Center's Cardiac Rehabilitation Program and San Diego State University's Exercise Physiology Laboratory and Adult Fitness Program.

Having researched exercise-related sudden death since 1981, Van Camp has written numerous articles and book chapters on the topic. He is on the editorial boards of both *Medicine and Science in Sports and Exercise* and *The Journal of Sports Medicine and Physical Fitness*. He also has been a reviewer for *The New England Journal of Medicine*, *The American Journal of Cardiology*, and *The Physician and Sportsmedicine*. Van Camp lectures around the world on nontraumatic sports death and the cardiovascular aspects of sports medicine.

Van Camp earned an MD from the UCLA School of Medicine in 1971. He is a Fellow of the ACSM, the American College of Cardiology, and the American Heart Association Council of Clinical Cardiology.